STRETCHING AND STRENGTHENING
FOR LOWER EXTREMITY AMPUTEES

Robert S. Gailey, Phd, P.T.
University of Miami, School of Medicine
Department of Orthopaedics and Rehabilitation
Division of Physical Therapy
Miami, Florida

Ann M. Gailey, M.S.P.T.

Illustrations by
Frank Angulo

An

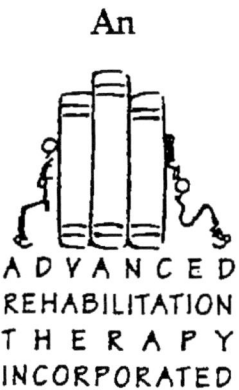

ADVANCED
REHABILITATION
THERAPY
INCORPORATED

Publication

All rights reserved. No part of this manual may be reproduced, stored in a retrieval system, or transmitted in any form or by any means, electronic, mechanical, photocopying, recorded, or otherwise, without written permission from the authors.

Copyright © 1994

Table of Contents

Introduction 1

Part I
Range of Motion and Stretching Exercise 5
Manual Stretching Program 9
Self-Stretching Program 13

Part II
Lower Extremity Strengthening Exercise 17
1. Isometric Strengthening 18
   Isometric Strengthening Program 19

2. Manual Resistance Strengthening 25
   Manual Strengthening Program 28

3. Isotonic Strengthening 38
   Isotonic Strengthening Program for Lower Extremities 41
   Isotonic Strengthening Program for Upper Extremities 49

4. Isokinetic Strengthening 56
   Isokinetic Strengthening Program 58

Introduction

Preparing an individual who has lost a lower limb for prosthetic training is conceptually no different than rehabilitating any other orthopedic patient. Applying the principles of functional progressive rehabilitation provides a well-rounded program which ensures that all of the neuromuscular and cardiorespiratory systems have been appropriately addressed.

Range of motion (ROM) and strengthening exercises are typically considered the foundation for all other skills and activities. Therefore, this monograph will address several methods of maintaining ROM and promoting strength. Although most forms of stretching and strengthening will be discussed briefly, it is important to keep in mind that many other exercises exist, and that the therapist must individualize every rehabilitation program for each patient.

The importance of maintaining adequate ROM and strength cannot be overemphasized with amputees of any age. The difference between becoming a household ambulator and returning to an active life style is frequently directly related to the ability to ambulate independently with a prosthesis. If the amputee is unable to maneuver the prosthesis comfortably, without exaggerated gait deviations, the incidence of rejection of the prosthesis, and in turn, the possibility of a premature sedentary lifestyle increases.

The most common limitations in ROM observed with specific levels of amputation include: flexion contracture alone, or a combination of flexion, abduction and external rotation with above-knee amputees. In the case of below-knee amputees, loss of extension at the knee is most frequently seen. Historically, a large number of the contractures seen were attributed to the surgical procedures where the severed muscle was left unattached, and as a result it retracted. With no attachment, or ability to generate a force, muscle imbalances occurred where the intact muscle group would pull the limb uncontested into a shortened position. For example: severed hamstrings were unable to apply sufficient force against the hip flexors resulting in hip flexion contractures, or retracted hip adductor muscles could not prevent hip abductor muscles from causing abduction contractures.

Today the universally accepted surgical procedures of myoplasty: suturing muscle to muscle, or myodesis: attaching muscle to bone, have significantly reduced the incidence of contractures related to muscle imbalances. However, that is not to say that the potential for loss of ROM no longer exists. If proper stretching exercises are not routinely performed, all amputees are at risk for losing ROM. Also, it must be kept in mind that shorter residual limbs at all levels of amputation are more prone to losses in ROM than limbs with greater length.

Any time a significant loss of ROM occurs, there is a direct effect on the prosthetic fit and on the gait pattern of the amputee. Limited modifications may be incorporated into the prosthesis in an attempt to minimize the effect that limited motion will have on the amputee's gait. Frequently, an acceptable result may be obtained, but rarely can prosthetic modifications restore normal joint function to a compromised anatomical joint. Table 1. highlights potential problems associated with the more commonly observed ROM limitations in amputees.

Table 1. Prosthetic Corrections and Gait Results When Joint Limitations are Present.

Position of Joint Limitation	Prosthetic Correction	Gait Result (If uncorrected)
Hip flexion	1. Greater initial hip flexion must be set into the socket.	1. Limited hip extension during late stance will result in a shorter stride length with the sound side. 2. Knee joint instability, often a result of joint position and in turn weak hip extension. 3. Increased lumbar lordosis during stance.
Hip abduction	1. Difficulty with weight bearing in the socket.	1. An abducted and/or circumducted gait. 2. Lateral bending of the trunk during stance.
Hip external rotation	1. A pelvic band with hip joint may be required to dampen rotational forces.	1. Medial whip during swing
Knee flexion	1. 15° contractures or less socket is set in greater flexion. 2. 15°-45° contractures are fitted with sockets set in greater flexion but they are less cosmetically appealing. 3. 45° contractures or greater, a bent knee prosthesis must be fabricated.	1. Uncorrected a foot flat gait pattern results. Socket correction permits heel contact at initial contact. 2. Foot flat gait pattern at initial contact and a shorter step with the prosthetic limb. 3. Essentially functions as a knee disarticulation gait, remaining in extension throughout stance without active knee flexion during swing.

The necessity for adequate strength in both the lower and upper extremities is an important factor when restoring the ability to achieve the most basic of tasks such as transfers, as well as perform the more demanding activities of ambulation, ascending stairs or even running.

The ability for the human body to adapt has always been an amazing wonder, especially when taking into account the level of function some individuals attain with decreased strength. Some amputees achieve reasonable success with a prosthesis without spending appreciable time in a strength training program. However, there exists a large population of amputees who have an express desire to obtain the optimal benefit from their prosthesis and to maximize their level of everyday activity. The most expedient way to enhance physical and prosthetic ability is to achieve a level of strength that will facilitate balance, coordination, agility, speed, endurance and, as a result, prosthetic control.

The absence of strength, like the loss of ROM, has consequences prosthetically during ambulation. Tables 2&3 outline some of the potential gait deviations that may occur during the various phases of gait as a result of muscle weakness.

Table 2. Below-Knee Gait Deviations as a Result of Muscle Weakness.

Phase of Gait	Muscle Weakness	Gait Deviation
1. Initial Contact	1. Weak knee extensors 2. General weakness	1. Excessive knee flexion 2. Foot rotation (most frequently external rotation)
2. Loading Response	1. Weak knee extensors	1. Excessive knee extension
3. Mid-Stance	1. General weakness	1. Inability to fully weight bear into the prosthesis
4. Terminal Stance	1. Weak hip or knee extensors	1. Drop off (premature knee flexion, prosthesis appears too short)
5. Pre-Swing	1. Weak hip extensors or abdominals	1. Increased lumbar lordosis
6. Initial Swing	1. Weak hip or knee flexors 2. Muscle atrophy	1. Toe drag or stubbing (inability to clear the floor) 2. Excessive pistoning within the socket
7. Mid-Swing	1. Weak hip or knee flexors 2. Weak knee or hip flexors and/or hip adductors	1. Vaulting on sound foot 2a. Circumducted gait 2b. Pelvic rise
8. General	1. General weakness	1a. Shortened stride length on the sound side 1b. Faster step with the sound limb 1c. Poor balance 1d. Uneven arm swing

Table 3. Above-Knee Gait Deviations as a Result of Muscle Weakness.

Phase of Gait	Muscle Weakness	Gait Deviation
1. Initial Contact	1. General weakness 2. Weak hip extensors	1. Foot rotation 2. Knee instability
2. Loading Response	none	none
3. Mid-Stance	1. Weak hip abductors, back extensors or abdominal 2. Weak hip adductors	1. Lateral bending of the trunk 2. Abducted gait
4. Terminal Stance	none	none
5. Pre-Swing	1. Weak hip extensors or abdominals	1. Increased lumbar lordosis
6. Initial Swing	1. General weakness	1a. Excessive pistoning within the socket 1b. Continuing whip (medial to lateral whip during swing)
7. Mid-Swing	1. Weak hip flexors 2. Weak hip flexors and/or adductors 3. Weak external rotators 4. Weak internal rotators	1. Vaulting on sound foot 2. Circumducted gait 3. Lateral whip 4. Medial whip
8. General	1. General weakness	1a. Shortened stride length on the sound side 1b. Faster step with the sound limb 1c. Poor balance 1d. Uneven arm swing

This monograph is part of a series designed as a complete amputee rehabilitation program. Gait training is not discussed in this manual as it has been discussed in detail in the manual entitled "Prosthetic Gait Training for Lower Extremity Amputees" by the same authors. This text is written to present exercises to two distinct readers: the amputee and the therapist. Independent exercises are written in lay terms for the amputee with spaces provided for the therapist to prescribe the cadence, repetitions, and sets for each exercise. The authors strongly recommend that the therapist review the exercises with the amputee to instruct appropriate form and to determine appropriate criteria for each exercise prescribed. Photocopies are permitted for pages that acknowledge permission, so that the amputee may have a copy to follow when performing a home exercise program. Exercises that require assistance are written in a therapeutic language specifically designed for the therapist. The authors do not expect the patient to perform these exercises at home with untrained assistance.

"The Rehabilitation Workbook for Lower Extremity Amputees" provides all the appropriate exercises from this series so that amputees may have a written guide to help them through the rehabilitation process.

PART I
Range of Motion and Stretching Exercises

Maintaining sufficient range of motion (ROM) has many benefits, including: enhancing performance, permitting joints to accommodate to stress and dissipate the impact of shock, and preventing muscle imbalances and injury. With age and reduced activity, loss of ROM is the expected norm. Unfortunately for amputees, the consequences of a significant reduction in ROM or, even worse, a contracture, may be a severely compromised prosthetic fit, gait and general function. This creates increased stress on other joints of the residual limb, the spine or the sound lower limb, when wearing the prosthesis. In some extreme cases, a contracture may eliminate the possibility of ambulation with a prosthesis altogether.

Fortunately, most limitations in joint movement severe enough to affect prosthetic fit are preventable when the therapist performs stretching or passive range of motion (PROM), regularly monitoring the amputee's joint motion. If loss of ROM occurs as a result of muscular shortening, manual stretching is one alternative employed to restore ROM. The frequency of PROM or manual stretching is individual to each amputee. Likewise, because there are many other rehabilitation services that require more of the therapist's expertise, educating the amputee to perform self-ROM, or stretching on a routine basis can help to maximize the efficiency of the time the therapist and patient spend together.

The following stretching exercise program presents two methods of exercise that will assist in maintaining or restoring joint motion: First, PROM or manual stretching performed by the therapist, or possibly, by a family member or friend educated by the therapist in the techniques; second, self-stretching performed independently by the amputee.

A third method of treatment for increasing joint ROM is passive joint mobilization. Joint mobilization should only be performed by a qualified therapist. There exists a vast body of information concerning joint mobilization by various authors discussing philosophy of treatment and technique. Suffice it to say that joint mobilization is an excellent means of promoting ROM and should be considered by the therapist when deciding alternatives for treatment.

General Instructions [24]

Regardless of the method of stretching used to increase ROM, some simple principles should be followed to ensure that maximum benefit is derived from each stretching session. The following list identifies some of the basic principles of flexibility and stretching:

1. Perform stretching exercises on a firm surface, in a room conducive to quiet, and wear loose comfortable clothing.

2. Relax and learn to become in touch with your body, avoiding tension in the muscle being stretched, or contractions of other muscles groups throughout the body.

3. Breathing must be regular and relaxed, avoiding breath holding and strained facial expressions.

4. Stretching must be slow, gentle and specific, avoiding quick ballistic stretching. (Ballistic stretching creates significantly more tension within the muscle being stretched, and for this reason is not appropriate for the majority of the amputee population.)

5. Each movement must be deliberate, with the emphasis placed on form rather than mobility, therefore avoiding unwanted substitutions of movement.

6. Avoid pain and discomfort that may lead to undesirable muscle contractions, substitutions, or soreness.

7. Do not force any movement beyond its normal ROM. Hyperflexibility should be avoided as it does not enhance function, and may lead to injury.

8. Increases in ROM obtained from one session may not carry over to the next. ROM achieved in one session should not be expected in the next session.

9. Avoid self-competition and competition with other individuals.

Warning: Any exercise activities not approved by appropriate medical personnel can have harmful results. Prior to starting any exercise program, have your doctor or therapist assess your medical and physical status. All exercise programs should be prescribed by a board-certified and registered professional. If, at any time, sudden pain or lasting discomfort should result, consult your doctor immediately.

Suggested Techniques:

Suggested techniques of PROM and stretching: The following is not intended to be a complete list of all the possible methods of PROM or stretching. Instead, it is designed to provide a few widely accepted techniques that have proven to be successful with a majority of the amputee population.

1. **Passive Range of Motion (PROM)**
   PROM is not a true stretching technique because the movement remains within the unrestricted available range, whereas stretching techniques take the joint past the available ROM in an attempt to increase the available ROM.

   a. Securely take hold of the appropriate limb segment and slowly move the joint to the comfortable limit of available motion without causing pain.
   b. Once at the end range, hold the limb for one to two seconds and return to the starting position slowly.
   c. A one to two second rest period at the starting position without releasing hand placement will be sufficient.
   d. When the prescribed number of repetitions have been completed, return to the resting position.

2. **Manual Passive Stretching**
   a. Securely take hold of the appropriate limb segment and slowly move the joint to the comfortable limit of available motion.
   b. Stretch the soft tissues of the joint by moving the limb past the limit of motion slowly, without causing pain.
   c. Hold the limb in the new position for a count of:
      10-15 seconds for beginners
      30-60 seconds for intermediate
      60-120 seconds for advanced
   Currently, the investigative literature does not identify any specific duration of stretch to be superior over another. Therefore, stretching to the individual's tolerance appears to be the most appropriate method.[16,24]
   d. At the completion of the stretch, return the limb to the comfortable limit of available joint motion, and rest for a pre-determined length of time. Typically, a 5-10 second rest period will be sufficient.
   e. When the prescribed number of repetitions has been completed, return to the resting position.

3. Contract-Relax or Hold-Relax Stretching [32,33]

a. Securely take hold of the appropriate limb segment and slowly move the joint to the comfortable limit of available motion.
b. Have the amputee contract the muscle group being stretched by:
   (1) actively contracting into the therapist's hands for the contract-relax technique
   or
   (2) meeting the resistance applied to the limb by the therapist for the hold-relax technique
   * No movement during the contraction should be permitted for either technique.
   * The duration of contraction for both techniques should be 6-10 seconds.
c. Pause for 1-2, seconds and allow the muscle to relax briefly after the contraction is completed.
d. Stretch the soft tissues of the joint by moving the limb past the limit of motion slowly, without causing pain.
e. Hold the limb in the new position for a count of:
   10-15 seconds for beginners
   30-60 seconds for advanced
f. At the completion of the stretch, keep the limb at the new limit of available joint motion and repeat the contract or hold procedure, pause and stretch.
g. When the prescribed number of repetitions have been completed return to the resting position. Small increments in range should be attempted with each repetition.

Variation:
Either the contract-relax or the hold-relax technique may incorporate a concentric contraction by the muscle group opposite to the muscle group being stretched. Theoretically, the tight muscle will relax as a result of reciprocal inhibition when the agonist muscle contracts concentrically. The contraction of the agonist muscle group should build slowly, avoiding any sudden movements that could injure the antagonistic muscle being stretched.

Note: The isometric contractions performed during any of the above techniques need not be maximal contractions. A sub-maximal contraction will suffice to inhibit the muscle group being stretched. A maximal contraction only creates more work for the therapist and tension within the muscle may continue after relaxation should occur.

1. PROM / Manual Passive / Contract-Relax (C-R) or Hold Relax (H-R) Stretching

1. Hip Flexor Stretch

a. Patient lies prone. A pillow may be placed under the hips to prevent low back strain.

b. Therapist passively extends the hip joint to the available range.
*If C-R or H-R is being used, have the patient perform the contraction now.

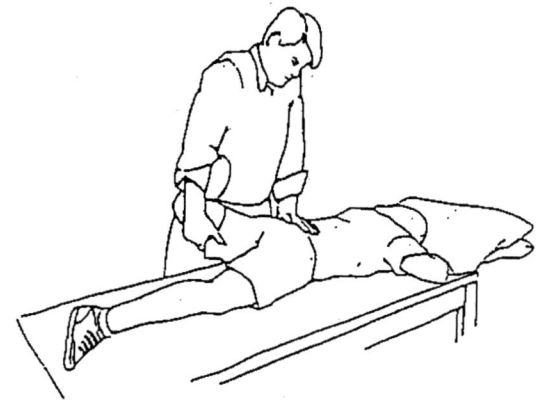

c. Move the limb into the new available range for a count of _____ seconds.

d. Relax the limb for a count of _____ seconds.

e. Repeat the exercise for _____ repetitions.

Primary muscles: rectus femoris, iliopsoas

2. Hip Abductor Stretch

a. Patient lies sidelying.

b. Therapist passively extends the hip joint and adducts the limb.
*If C-R or H-R is being used, have the patient perform the contraction now.

c. Move the limb into the new available range for a count of _____ seconds.

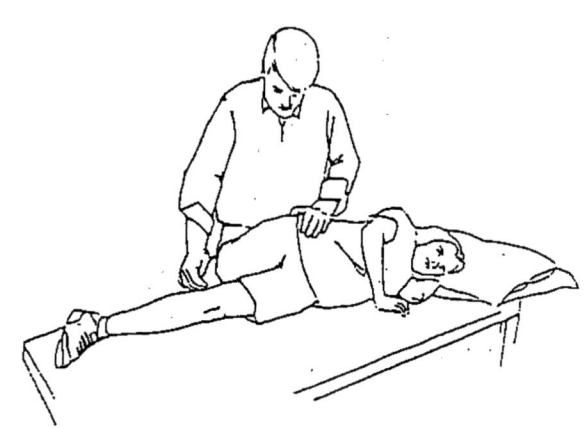

d. Relax the limb for a count of _____ seconds.

e. Repeat the exercise for _____ repetitions.

Primary muscles: gluteus medius, gluteus minimus

3. Hip Adductor Stretch

a. Patient lies supine.

b. Therapist passively abducts the hip joint.
   *If C-R or H-R is being used, have the patient perform the contraction now.

c. Move the limb into the new available range for a count of _____ seconds.

d. Relax the limb for a count of _____ seconds.

e. Repeat the exercise for _____ repetitions.

Primary muscles: adductor magnus, adductor longus, adductor brevis, gracilis

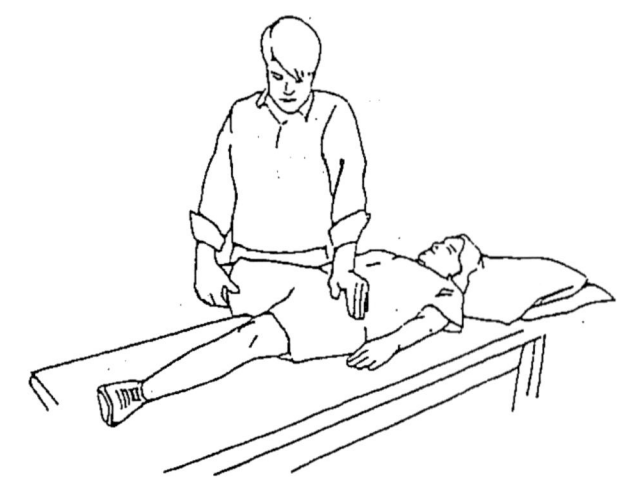

4. Hip Extensor Stretch

a. Patient lies supine.

b. Therapist passively flexes the hip joint while the knee joint remains flexed.
   *If C-R or H-R is being used, have the patient perform the contraction now.

c. Move the limb into the new available range for a count of _____ seconds.

d. Relax the limb for a count of _____ seconds.

e. Repeat the exercise for _____ repetitions.

Primary muscles: gluteus maximus, hamstrings

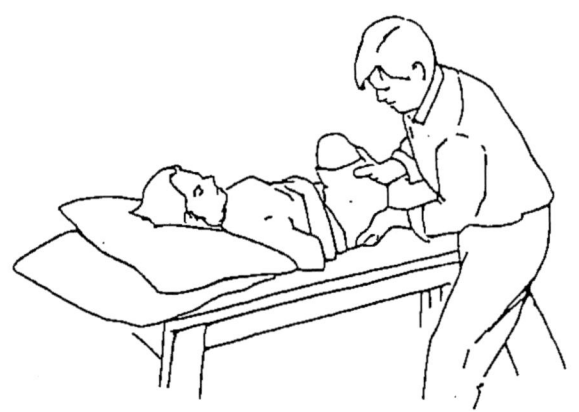

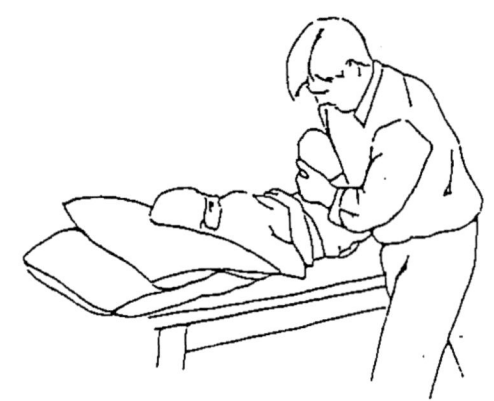

5. Hip Abductor/External Rotator Stretch

a. Patient lies supine.

b. Therapist passively flexes the hip joint and adducts the limb diagonally across the patient's chest.
*If C-R or H-R is being used, have the patient perform the contraction now.

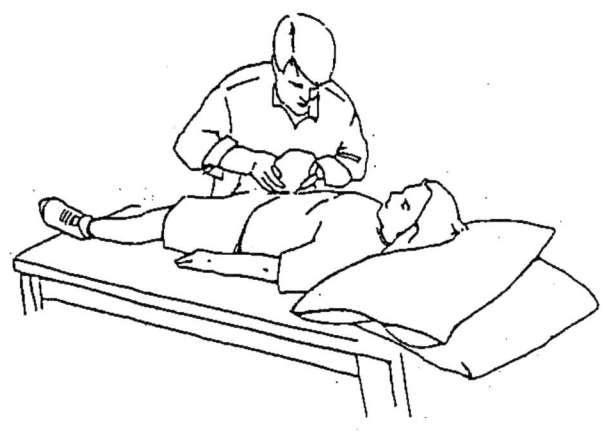

c. Move the limb into the new available range for a count of _____ seconds.

d. Relax the limb for a count of _____ seconds.

e. Repeat the exercise for _____ repetitions.

Variation: flex the hip and knee 90 degrees while supporting the knee internally or externally

Primary muscles: gluteus medius, gluteus minimus, piriformis

6. Knee Extensor Stretch

a. Patient lies prone.

b. Therapist passively flexes the knee joint to available range.
*If C-R or H-R is being used, have the patient perform the contraction now.

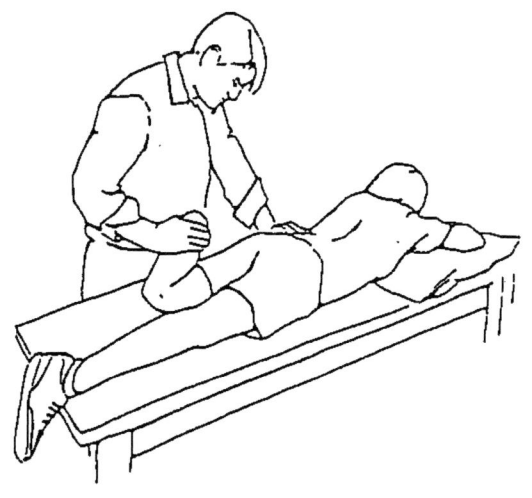

c. Move the limb into the new available range for a count of _____ seconds.

d. Relax the limb for a count of _____ seconds.

e. Repeat the exercise for _____ repetitions.

Primary muscles: quadriceps group

Variation: Therapist flexes hip and knee passively with patient supine.

7. Knee Flexor Stretch

a. Patient lies supine.

b. Therapist passively extends knee joint to full extension and flexes hip joint to available range.
*If C-R or H-R is being used, have the patient perform the contraction now.

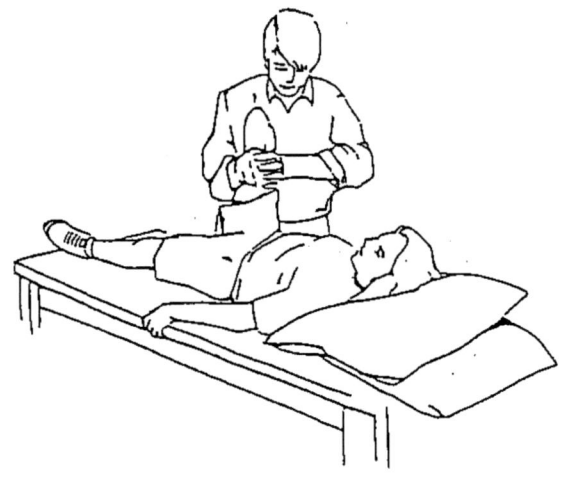

c. Move the limb into the new available range for a count of _____ seconds.

d. Relax the limb for a count of _____ seconds.

e. Repeat the exercise for _____ repetitions.

Primary muscles: hamstrings

2. Self-Stretching

Warning: Any exercise activities not approved by appropriate medical personnel can have harmful results. Prior to starting any exercise program, have your doctor or therapist assess your medical and physical status. All exercise programs should be prescribed by a board-certified and registered professional. If, at any time, sudden pain or lasting discomfort should result, consult your doctor immediately.

General Instructions

a. Assume the resting or starting position as described.

b. Slowly move the limb to the comfortable limit of the available joint motion.

c. Stretch the soft tissues of the joint by moving past the limit of available motion slowly without causing pain.

d. Hold the new position for a count of:

    10-15 seconds for beginners
    30-60 seconds for intermediate
    60-120 seconds for advanced

Currently, the investigative literature does not identify any specific duration of stretch to be superior over another. Therefore, stretching to the individual's tolerance appears to be the most appropriate method.

e. At the completion of the stretch, return to the comfortable limit of available motion and rest for a pre-determined length of time. Typically, a 5-10 second rest period will be sufficient.

f. When the prescribed number of repetitions have been completed, return to the resting position.

g. No stretch should be performed to the point of pain.

1. Hip Flexor Stretch

   a. Lie comfortably on your stomach with both legs straight.

   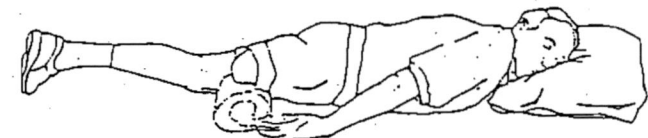

   b. Place a towel roll under your residual limb. The height of the towel roll should promote a stretch. (Below-knee amputees should extend the support from just above the knee to the end of the residual limb. No pressure should be on the knee cap.)

   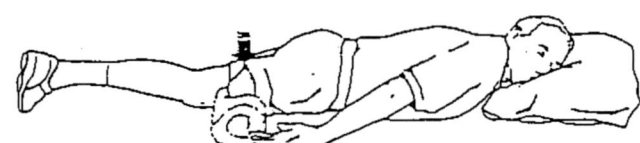

   c. Hold the stretched position for a count of _____ seconds.

   d. Return to the starting position and relax the limb for a count of _____ seconds.

   e. Repeat for _____ repetitions, performing _____ sets.

   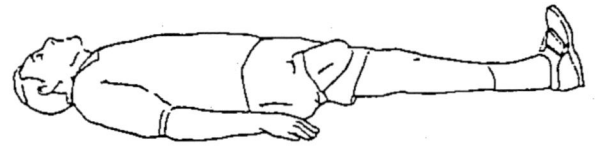

   Primary muscles: rectus femoris, iliopsoas

2. Hip Extensor Stretch

   a. Lie comfortably on your back with both legs straight.

   b. Bend your hip so that your residual limb or bent knee moves toward your chest.

   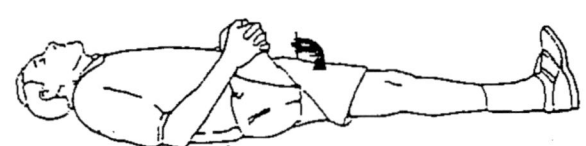

   c. Hold the stretched position for a count of _____ seconds.

   d. Return to the starting position and relax the limb for a count of _____ seconds.

   e. Repeat for _____ repetitions, performing _____ sets.

   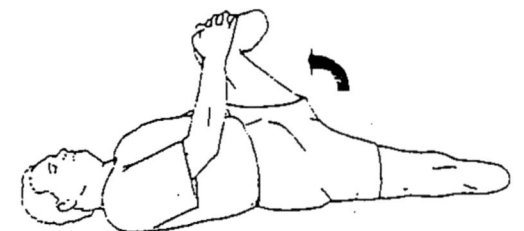

   Primary muscles: gluteus maximus, hamstrings

3. Hip Abductor/Extensor Rotator Stretch

a. Lie comfortably on your back with both legs straight.

b. Bend your hip so that your residual limb or bent knee moves toward your opposite shoulder.

c. Hold the stretched position for _____ seconds.

d. Return to the starting position and relax the limb for a count of _____ seconds.

e. Repeat for _____ repetitions, performing _____ sets.

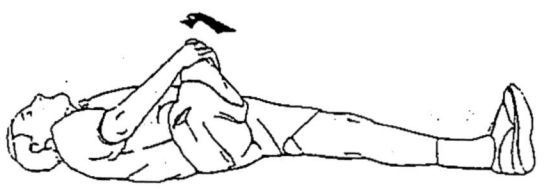

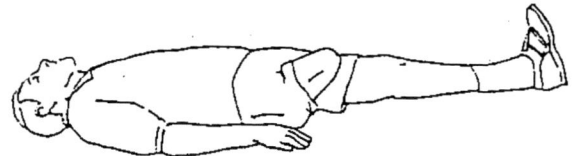

Primary muscles: gluteus medius, gluteus minimus, piriformis

4. Hip Adductor Stretch

a. Sit on a firm surface with legs straight.

b. Keep one leg stationary, spread your other leg as wide as possible using one hand to assist you, while the other hand provides support.

c. Hold the stretched position for a count of _____ seconds.

d. Return to the starting position and relax the limb for a count of _____ seconds.

e. Repeat for _____ repetitions, performing _____ sets.

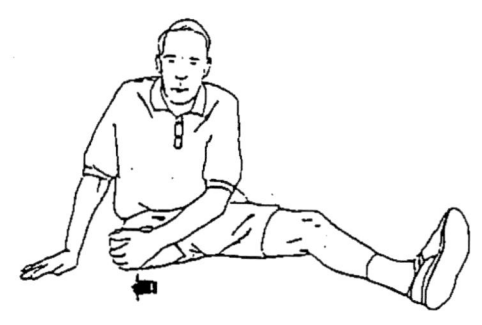

Primary muscles: adductor magnus, adductor longus, adductor brevis, gracilis

5. Knee Extensor Stretch

   a. Lie comfortably on your back with both legs straight.

   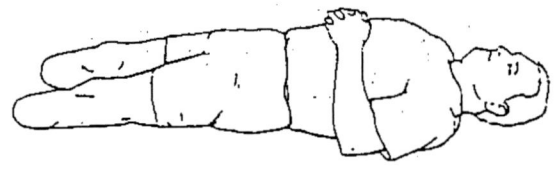

   b. Bend your hip, bringing your knee toward your chest. Grasp your leg below the knee and bend your knee to the appropriate limit of motion.

   c. Hold the stretched position for a count of _____ seconds.

   d. Return to the starting position and relax the limb for a count of _____ seconds.

   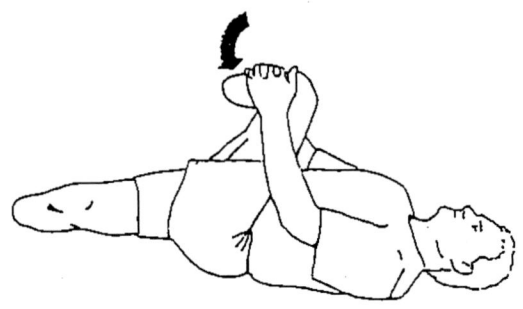

   e. Repeat for _____ repetitions, performing _____ sets.

   Primary muscles: vastus lateralis, medius, and intermedius (the rectus femoris is not stretched during this exercise)

   Note: The rectus femoris will not receive a stretch as it crosses the hip.

6. Knee Flexor Stretch

   a. Sit on a firm surface, with legs apart, and knees extended.

   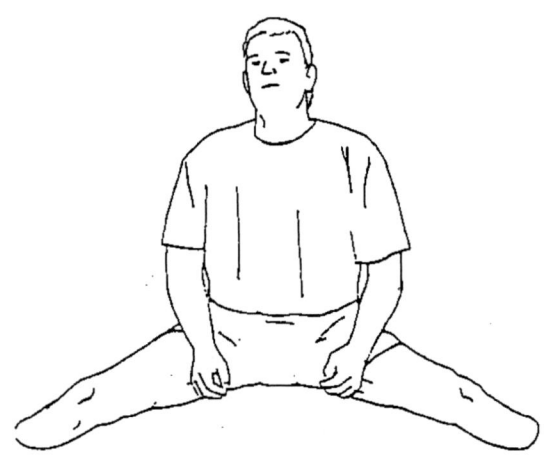

   b. Reaching arms forward and keeping trunk erect, lean your chest toward your thigh until a stretch is felt in the back of the leg.

   c. Hold the stretched position for a count of _____ seconds.

   d. Raise your trunk and relax for a count of _____ seconds.

   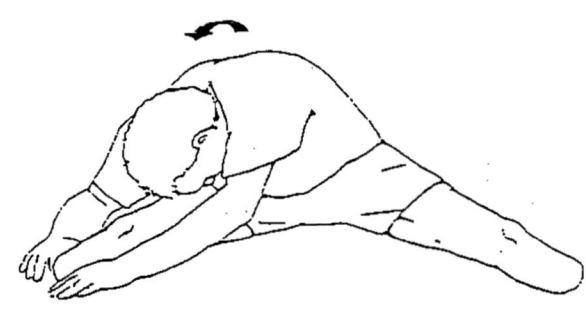

   e. Repeat for _____ repetitions, performing _____ sets.

   Primary muscles: hamstrings

PART II
Lower Extremity Strengthening Exercises

Strengthening is one of the most important precursors to achieving many of the skills required in transfers, functional skills, and ambulation. The selection of the type of strengthening exercise is dependent upon a variety of factors. For example, initial muscular strength and endurance, level of independence, access to equipment, time constraints, safety, and several other issues all play a significant role in determining what methods of strengthening are best for a particular individual during a specific stage of rehabilitation.

In most instances, people are progressed through several methods of strengthening as they move through the rehabilitation process. For example, the amputee may initially be taught isometrics, the safest and most independent form of strengthening when first recovering from a major surgery. As strength and general mobility improve, isotonics (without any resistance), commonly referred to as active exercises, are instructed. As the individual's strength increases with time and practice, some form of resistance is added so that a program of progressive resistive exercise (PREs) is formulated. After a baseline of strength is developed, some amputees will benefit from a highly specialized form of strengthening called isokinetics. Isokinetics require expensive, technical equipment that allows the individual to strengthen a body segment at different speeds, which may be important for certain amputees.

Most importantly, every amputee should be taught a strengthening program which will continue the strengthening process after discharge from the rehabilitation center, fostering a level of fitness that will allow a quality physical lifestyle. This requires the transition from exercising in a sterile clinical environment, which is often perceived as a place where the sick and debilitated meet, to a general health facility such as a club or fitness center. By introducing the amputee to the principles of fitness, and instructing a PRE program that is easily transferable to any environment, the transition from rehabilitation to everyday life can be realized. If possible, introducing the amputee to a fitness center close to their home is an excellent method of mainstreaming them back to the community.

The following is an overview of several methods of strengthening, specific to the amputee. As with all strengthening programs, some exercises may need to be varied according to the individual needs of each amputee. The program suggested is not all-inclusive and there are many different exercises available that extend beyond the scope of this text. However, the exercises identified are beneficial for the majority of amputees of all ages, and are believed to be a good beginner-to-intermediate strengthening program.

1. Isometrics [7, 8, 10, 19, 24, 25]

Isometric exercises require a muscular contraction where there is no appreciable change in length of the muscle. In other words, the muscle neither shortens nor lengthens and no movement results, therefore, the joint angle remains unchanged. The isometric program presented is a variation of Eibert and Tester's (1956) "Dynamic Stump Exercises."

Advantages:
1. Good introductory activity for atrophied or disused muscles. An excellent exercise to teach bedside.
2. The safest form of strengthening, as no equipment is required.
3. Can be performed anywhere.
4. Can be performed during limb immobilization.
5. Maintains strength of degenerative joints with reduced possibility of inflaming arthritic joints.

Disadvantages:
1. Potentially the least effective form of strength improvement once muscle strength progresses past the initial stages.
2. Increased hypertension experience, therefore appropriate breathing patterns during exercise are important.
3. There is no increase in joint ROM, and strength is primarily developed at the joint angle at which the exercise is performed, with a physiological overflow of 20 degrees, ten degrees in each direction from the angle of resistance.[25]
4. Muscular endurance is not developed as well as in other forms of strengthening.
5. Muscular coordination, agility, and other synergistic movements necessary for functional activities are not promoted.

Equipment:
1. Towel roll of 5-7 inches in thickness.
2. A foot stool of 7 inches in height.
3. A large, firm resting surface such as a floor or exercise mat.
4. Loose comfortable clothing, i.e. shorts and a T-shirt.

Warning: Any exercise activities not approved by appropriate medical personnel can have harmful results. Prior to starting any exercise program, have your doctor or therapist assess your medical and physical status. All exercise programs should be prescribed by a board-certified and registered professional. If, at any time, sudden pain or lasting discomfort should result, consult your doctor immediately.

General Instructions:

Each repetition should be performed for 10 seconds. This will allow you to perform each repetition slowly, moving your body in a controlled manner.[7]

2 sec. initiate contraction (raising the body)
6 sec. maintain the contraction (hold the position)
<u>2 sec. release contraction (lowering the body)</u>
10 sec. total time of each repetition

Note: A 10 second contraction may be too difficult to maintain initially. You may begin with a 6 second repetition by decreasing holding time to 2 seconds.

2 sec. initial contraction
2 sec. maintain the contraction
<u>2 sec. release contraction</u>
6 sec. total time

1. Progress to 10 second repetitions when possible.

2. Between each repetition, a 5-10 second rest period is recommended to allow the muscle ample time to recover in order to perform the next repetition correctly.

3. If possible, add 5 repetitions each week, up to 20-30 repetitions.

4. Perform each of these exercises twice a day for four weeks or until you can perform 20-30 repetitions for 10 seconds each with correct form.

5. Once you are able to perform 25 repetitions correctly, you may perform these exercises once a day for eight weeks or make them a part of your daily exercise program.

6. Typically, individuals who are able to perform 25 isometric repetitions correctly should move on to isotonic progressive resistive exercises (PRE). However, for those individuals who do not have access to equipment, nor wish to perform a PRE strengthening program, continuation of the isometric program is appropriate.

Program Example:
(10 sec. contraction + 10 sec. rest) x 10 repetitions = 3 min. 20 sec.
7 exercises x 3 min. 20 sec. = 23 min. 20 sec. per session

Note: As your strength and endurance increase, less rest between repetitions will be needed, thus decreasing the total exercise session time.

1. Hip Extension

   a. Lie on your back with the towel/stool placed securely under the residual limb. Both arms rest comfortably at your sides.

   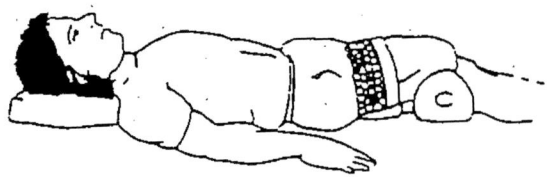

   b. Depress the residual limb firmly into the towel/stool, raising your buttocks off the resting surface.

   c. Hold this position for ____ seconds, then lower your buttocks slowly to the resting position.

   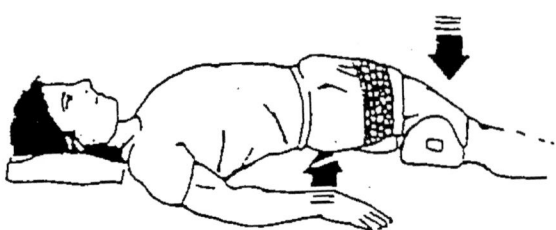

   d. Repeat this exercise for ____ repetitions.

   Variation: As your strength increases, raise the unaffected limb off the resting surface throughout the exercise. Additional resistance may be provided by resting a weight on the pelvis.

   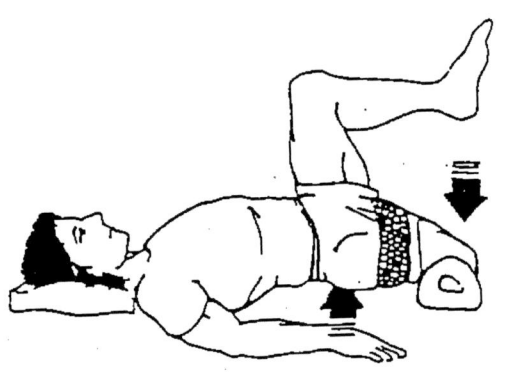

   Primary muscles: gluteals and hamstrings

2. Hip Abduction

   a. Lie on the affected limb side with the towel/stool placed securely under the residual limb. Place a stool directly in front of your hips, bending both your unaffected hip and knee to 90 degrees so that the leg rests comfortably on the stool.

   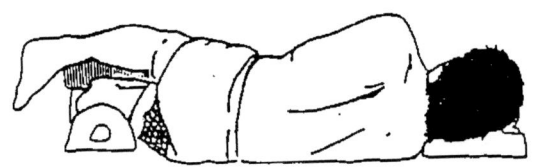

   b. Depress the residual limb firmly into the towel/stool, raising your hip off the resting surface.

   c. Hold this position for ____ seconds, then lower yourself slowly back to the resting position.

   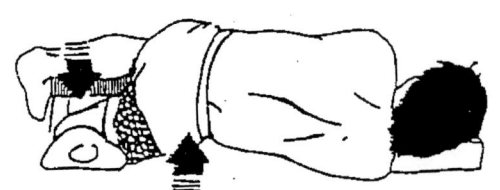

   d. Repeat this exercise for ____ repetitions.

Variation: As your strength increases, begin to lift the unaffected limb off the stool, maintaining leg in an outstretched position held directly over the residual limb. Additional resistance may be achieved by resting a weight on the sound hip.

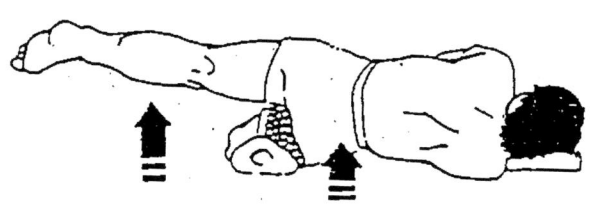

Primary muscles: gluteus medius and gluteus minimus

3. Hip Flexion

a. Lie on your stomach with the towel placed securely under the residual limb. Both arms should rest comfortably at your sides.

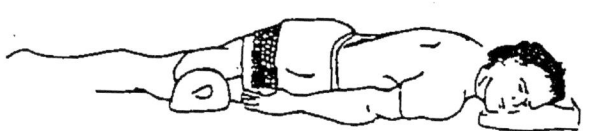

b. Depress the residual limb firmly into the towel raising pelvis off the resting surface.

c. Hold this position for _____ seconds, then lower yourself back to the resting position.

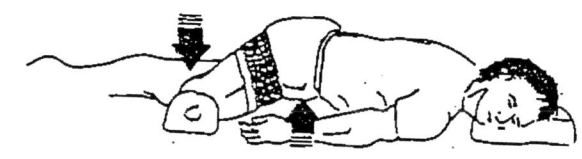

d. Repeat this exercise for _____ repetitions.

Variation: Additional resistance may be achieved by resting a weight on the buttocks.

Primary muscles: iliopsoas and rectus femoris

4. Back Extension

a. Lie on your stomach with a towel placed between your legs. Cross your arms behind your back.

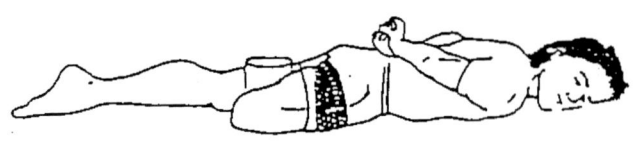

b. Squeeze the towel between your legs while simultaneously raising both legs, and head off the resting surface.

c. Hold this position for ____ seconds, then lower yourself back to the resting position.

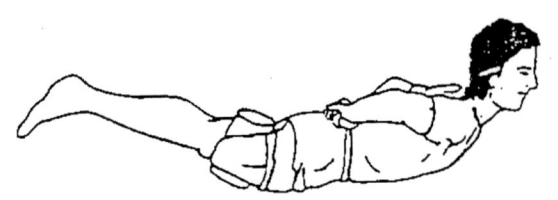

d. Repeat this exercise for ____ repetitions.

Variation: As your strength increases, begin raising more of your upper body off the mat.

Primary muscles: back extensors, gluteus maximus and hip adductors

5. Hip Adduction

a. Lie on the unaffected side, placing the stool over the unaffected limb. Place your residual limb on top of the stool, covering the stool with a pillow for comfort. Place the lower arm under your head, and the upper arm comfortably at your side.

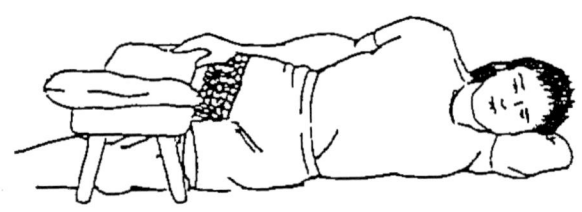

b. Depress the residual limb into the pillow-covered stool raising the lower hip off the resting surface.

c. Hold this position for ____ seconds, and then lower yourself back to the resting position.

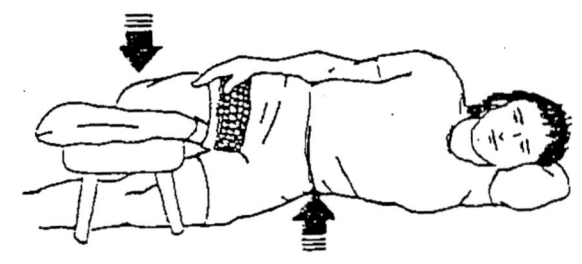

d. Repeat this exercise for ____ repetitions.

Variation: As your strength increases, raise your unaffected leg off the mat.

Primary muscles: hip adductors

6. Bridging

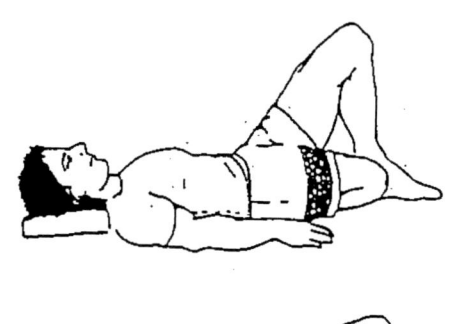

a. Lie on your back with the unaffected knee bent to 90 degrees and your foot flat on the resting surface. Place both arms comfortably by your sides.

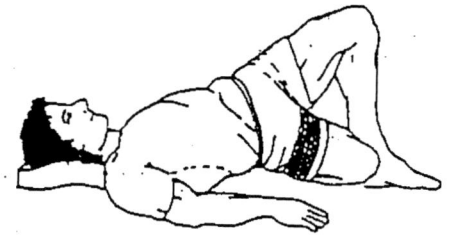

b. Push down with your foot into the resting surface, while raising your buttocks, until your hips are fully extended. Rotate the affected hip in an upward direction until both hips are of equal height.

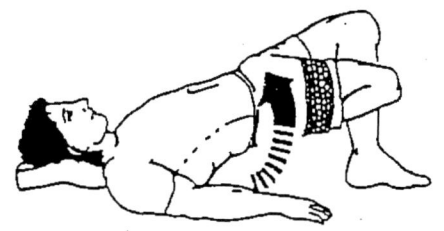

c. Hold this position for _____ seconds, and then lower yourself to the resting position.

d. Repeat this exercise for _____ repetitions.

Primary muscles: gluteus maximus, back extensors, unaffected side internal rotators

7. Sit-Ups

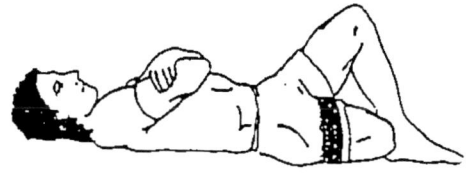

a. Lie on your back, arms across your chest and your knee bent.

b. Start with your head on the resting surface, tuck your chin and raise your trunk until your shoulder blades come off the resting surface.

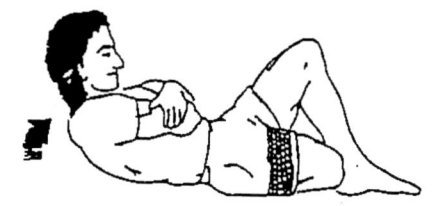

c. Hold this position for _____ seconds, and then lower yourself to the resting position.

d. Repeat this exercise for _____ repetitions.

Variation: As your strength increases begin to bring your knee to your chest as you raise your upper body off the resting surface.

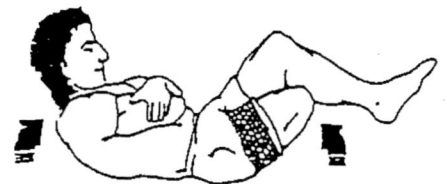

Primary muscles: abdominals

8. Knee Extension

   a. Lie on your stomach with a pillow placed securely under the residual limb thigh and another towel under the shin. The knee cap should not be touching the resting surface or the towels, so no compression occurs. Both arms rest comfortably.

   b. Depress the shin of the residual limb firmly into the towel extending the knee completely.

   c. Hold this position for _____ seconds, then relax the limb while returning to the resting position.

   d. Repeat this exercise for _____ repetitions.

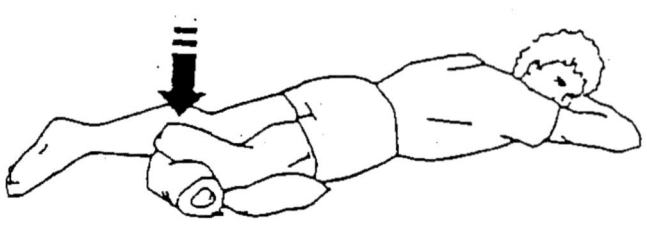

Primary muscles: quadriceps femoris

9. Knee Flexion

   a. Lie on your back with a firm towel roll placed under the calf of the residual limb. Both arms rest comfortably.

   b. Pull down and back into the towel roll as your knee begins to partially bend. The towel should not slide, if it does place additional towels under your thigh to prevent slipping.

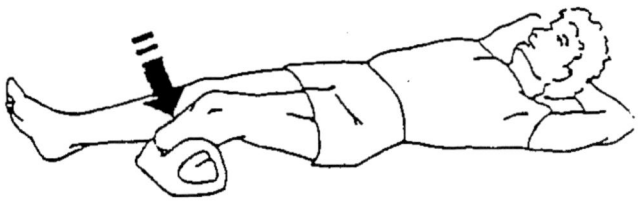

   c. Hold this position for _____ seconds, and then relax the limb while returning to the resting position.

   d. Repeat this exercise for _____ repetitions.

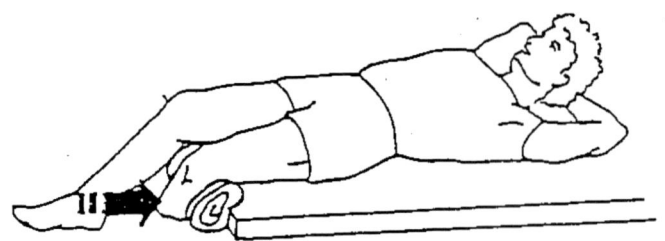

Variation: For a firmer surface lie on a table with the knee bent over the end of the table and pull your leg into the table.

Primary Muscles: hamstrings

2. Manual Resistance Strengthening Exercises [24, 32, 33]

Manual resistance exercise is an active resistance exercise requiring an accommodating physical force that is applied by a skilled therapist, producing either a dynamic or static contraction.[24]

Advantages:
1. Two types of muscular contractions (isometric and isotonic) may be performed.
2. Graded resistance may be applied throughout the available range of motion.
3. Exercises may be performed in the anatomical planes or diagonal patterns.
4. Greater control of movement, with specific muscles strengthened as desired by the therapist.
5. No equipment is necessary.

Disadvantages:
1. Exercises must be performed by an experienced therapist.
2. There is no means to accurately quantify the amount of resistance being applied throughout the range of motion.
3. In some cases, strength gains are limited by the therapist's strength or ability to provide a biomechanical advantage.

Equipment:
1. A large, firm resting surface such as a plinth or mat table.
2. Loose, comfortable clothing. i.e. shorts and a T-shirt.

General Instructions:

1. Perform manual strengthening exercises on a safe, comfortable surface that permits both the patient and therapist to assume good working body mechanics.
2. Both the patient and therapist should breath normally and avoid breath holding and strained facial expressions.
3. Therapist hand placements are dependent upon the patient's strength, stability, and the direction of movement desired.
4. As a general rule, resistance should not be applied across two joints. However, if this is necessary, the middle joint must be stable and pain-free throughout the exercise.
5. Joints proximal to the exercised joint must be secure, therefore allowing maximum effort by the patient when required.
6. Graded resistance must be applied by the therapist throughout the range of motion, at a level of intensity that will permit the patient to complete the desired number of repetitions for each set.

Suggested Techniques:

1. Manual Resistance in Anatomical Planes
   Manual resistance in the anatomical planes follows the general instructions previously outlined. The application of this technique requires that the amputee be placed in a position where the therapist can resist the limb segment, as a single joint moves throughout the available range of motion in one plane. This technique is favored when a specific muscle, or muscle group requires particular attention. This technique is very effective and widely used, and the individual exercises are universally known by therapists. Numerous publications offer excellent illustrations and descriptions of the techniques available for every joint segment. As a result, these exercises will be omitted from this text.

2. Manual Resistance in Diagonal Patterns
   Manual resistance in diagonal patterns has become synonymous with the widely accepted method of Proprioceptive Neuromuscular Facilitation (PNF), which was first introduced by Dr. Herman Kabat, Margaret "Maggie" Knott and Dorothy Voss in the 1950s. Simply, but impeccably, stated: Techniques of PNF are used to place specific demands in order to secure a desired response.[33] Specific diagonal or spiral patterns were developed and combined with nine different facilitation techniques to create a method of rehabilitation that has proven to be extremely beneficial for all who correctly employ PNF techniques.

   PNF techniques have been demonstrated to be very worthwhile with amputees, not only to strengthen the intact limbs, but as a method of re-educating the residual limb in the synergistic movements necessary for prosthetic control during ambulation and other functional skills. Rotational and mass patterns for the trunk and pelvic musculature help to facilitate differentiation between the upper and lower body segments. The ability to develop adequate differentiation between the pelvis and trunk permits smoother contralateral trunk movement and arm swing during walking.

   For congenital and pediatric amputees, the introduction of pelvic and trunk patterns is essential for developing optimal gait mechanics. Frequently, congenital amputees fail to learn rotational movements as a result of the absent limb. Once initiated through therapy, children easily adopt the more natural movement patterns, and incorporate these learned skills into their gait and most other activities.

   To discuss the concepts, principles, or techniques of PNF in this text's format would never serve justice to the reader, or those rehabilitation pioneers who worked so hard to establish them. Likewise, it is strongly suggested that only those therapists who have received appropriate training employ PNF techniques.

   The following illustrations and brief descriptions that accompany the techniques are provided soley as memory joggers for therapists who typically use PNF as a rehabilitation tool. Keep in mind that manual contacts will vary depending on the desired movement, component of motion being emphasized, patient and therapist body mechanics and size, and range-limiting factors. As always, every patient should be evaluated for their individual needs and treated accordingly.

Philosophy

Mobility is the capability to initiate and maintain adequate movement throughout a functional range of motion, whereas stability is the ability to generate co-contraction about a joint sufficient enough to maintain weight-bearing and nonweight-bearing postures acceptable to the mid-line position. Facilitation of mobility and stability are promoted through various PNF techniques designed specifically for each function. For example, rhythmic initiation (a passive, repetitive movement throughout the desired ROM) and slow-reversal (isotonic contractions in one diagonal pattern with changes in direction performed alternately at the end of range) techniques promote mobility. While rhythmic stabilization (simultaneous isometric contraction of antagonists: co-contraction) and approximation (compression of joint surfaces) assist in developing postural stability.[32,33]

The development of the proximal musculature of the trunk, pelvis and shoulder girdle in amputees provides several benefits: 1) Typically, the trunk musculature of the amputee is in the fair to good range. Therefore, strengthening via trunk patterns will assist in facilitating strength increases through overflow to the weakened extremity musculature. 2) Strengthening of the trunk and pelvic musculature can enhance balance and decrease postural deficits brought about as a result of the amputation. 3) Providing the amputee with proximal stability of the trunk, pelvis, and shoulder girdle, which perform gross movements that require greater strength, will support mobility of the distal extremity musculature that is required for more refined skills. Pelvic motions initiate and advance the lower limb, while more distal musculature around the knee assists in accurate foot placement. If the knee is absent, the hip musculature must further develop the ability to correctly position the prosthetic foot.

Some of the patterns illustrated in this text are variations of the patterns discussed in other PNF publications. These patterns permit amputees to develop the required proximal musculature in positions that do not initially require quadruped or kneeling postures that are frequently difficult for them to assume. However, assistive equipment such as bolsters and wedges have often proven to be very effective in assisting amputees to be positioned correctly throughout the developmental sequence. The manual entitled "Balance, Agility, Coordination, and Endurance for Lower Extremity Amputees" by the same authors will illustrate some sitting, quadruped, kneeling and standing techniques for promoting stability.

Pelvic, Shoulder Girdle, and Trunk Patterns

Pattern: Pelvic Anterior Elevation

a. Position:
   Patient lies sidelying with hips and knees flexed to 90°.

b. Manual contacts:
   Both hands form a lumbrical grip over the anterior, superior iliac crest.

c. Motion:
   Pelvis - anterior, superior, elevation.

d. Command:
   "Pull, up and forward."

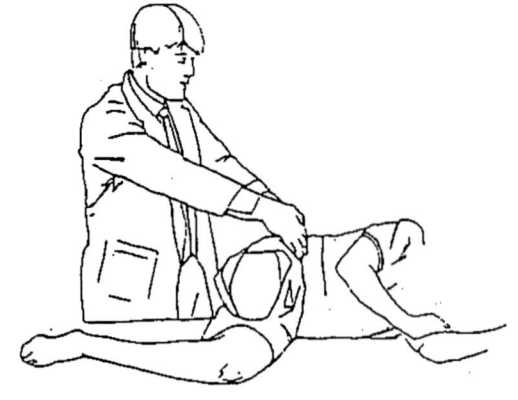

Pattern: Pelvic Posterior Depression

a. Position:
   Patient lies sidelying with hips and knees flexed to 90°.

b. Manual contacts:
   Both hands cup the ischial tuberosity.

c. Motion:
   Pelvis - posterior, inferior, depression.

d. Command:
   "Sit back into my hands."

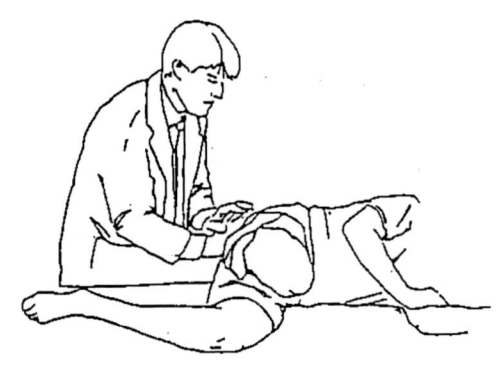

Pattern: Pelvic Anterior Depression

a. Position:
   Patient lies sidelying with hips and knees flexed to 90°.

b. Manual contacts:
   Posterior hand - ischial tuberosity.
   Anterior hand - ASIS

c. Motion:
   Pelvis - anterior, inferior, depression.

d. Command:
   "Pull, down and forward."

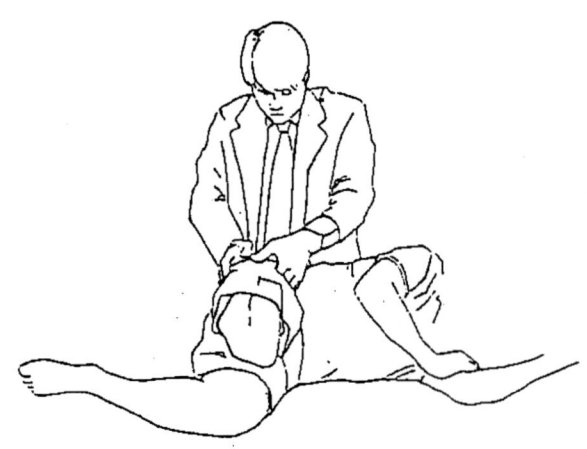

Pattern: Pelvic Posterior Elevation

a. Position:
Patient lies sidelying with hips and knees flexed to 90°.

b. Manual contacts:
Both hands form a lumbrical grip over the iliac crest.

c. Motion:
Pelvis - posterior, superior, elevation.

d. Command:
"Push, up and back."

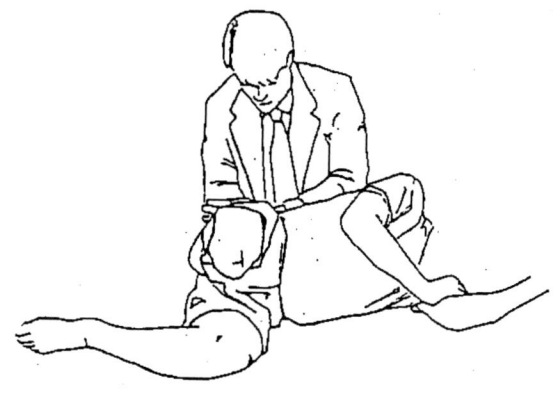

Pattern: Shoulder Girdle Anterior Elevation

a. Position:
Patient lies sidelying with hips and knees flexed to 90°, arms relaxed comfortably.

b. Manual contacts:
Both hands form a lumbrical grip over the anterior deltoid region.

c. Motion:
shoulder girdle - anterior, superior, elevation.

d. Command:
"Pull, up and forward."

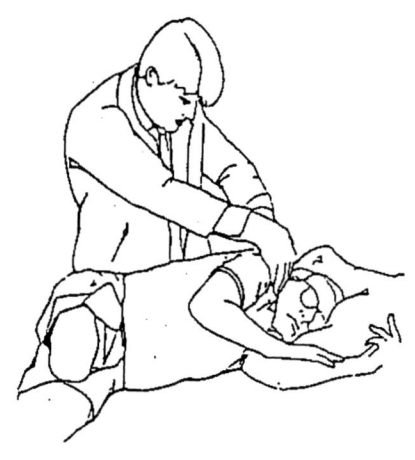

Pattern: Shoulder Girdle Posterior Depression

a. Position:
Patient lies sidelying with hips and knees flexed to 90°, arms relaxed comfortably.

b. Manual contacts:
Both hands cup the distal, medial aspect of the inferior angle of the scapula.

c. Motion:
shoulder girdle - posterior, inferior, depression.

d. Command:
"Push down and back into my hands."

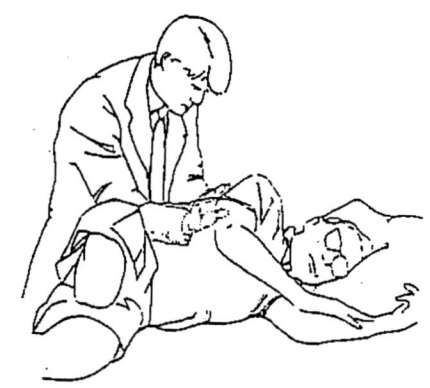

Pattern: Shoulder Girdle Anterior Depression

a. Position:
Patient lies sidelying with hips and knees flexed to 90°, arms relaxed comfortably.

b. Manual contacts:
Anterior hand - anterior aspect of the axilla.
Posterior hand - posterior aspect of the axilla.

c. Motion:
Shoulder girdle - anterior, inferior, depression.

d. Command:
"Pull, down and forward."

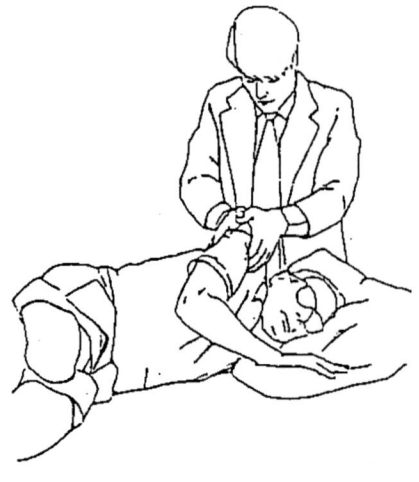

Pattern: Shoulder Girdle Posterior Elevation

a. Position:
Patient lies sidelying with hips and knees flexed to 90°, arms relaxed comfortably.

b. Manual contacts:
Both hands form a lumbrical grip over the posterior, superior deltoid region.

c. Motion:
Shoulder girdle - posterior, superior, elevation.

d. Command:
"Push, up and back into my hands."

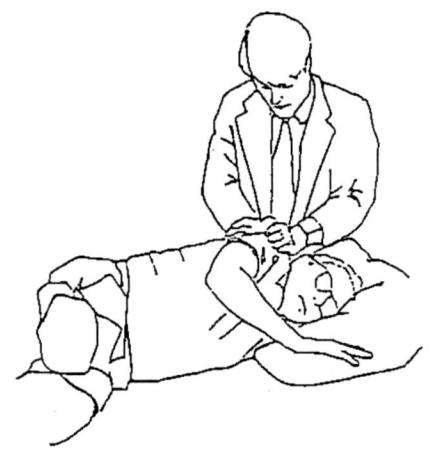

Pattern: Mass Trunk Flexion

a. Position:
Patient lies sidelying with hips and knees flexed to 90°, arms relaxed comfortably.

b. Manual contacts:
Distal hand - anterior superior iliac crest.
Proximal hand - lateral aspect of the deltoid (if possible the thumb and little finger anchor at the axilla).

c. Motion:
Trunk - flexion
Shoulder girdle - anterior depression
Pelvis - anterior elevation

d. Command:
"Curl into my hands."

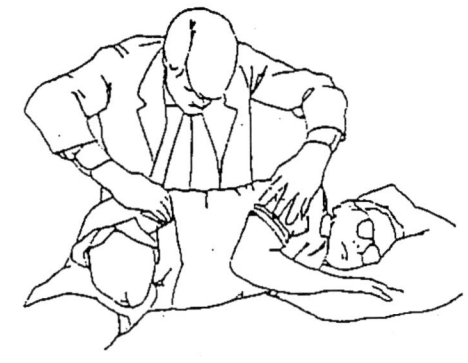

Pattern: Mass Trunk Extension

a. Position:
Patient lies sidelying with hips and knees flexed to 90°, arms relaxed comfortably.

b. Manual contacts:
Distal hand - ischial tuberosity.
Proximal hand - superior, posterior aspect of the deltoid.

c. Motion:
Trunk - Extension
Shoulder girdle - posterior elevation
Pelvis - posterior depression

d. Command:
"Push back into my hands."

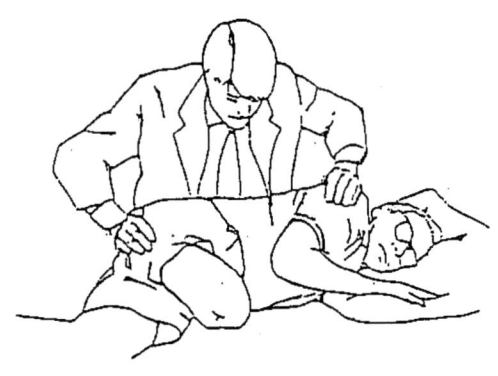

Pattern: Posterior Trunk Rotation

a. Position:
Patient lies sidelying with hips and knees flexed to 90°, arms relaxed comfortably.

b. Manual contacts:
Distal hand - anterior superior iliac crest.
Proximal hand - superior, posterior aspect of the deltoid.

c. Motion:
Trunk - posterior rotation
Shoulder girdle - posterior elevation
Pelvis - anterior elevation

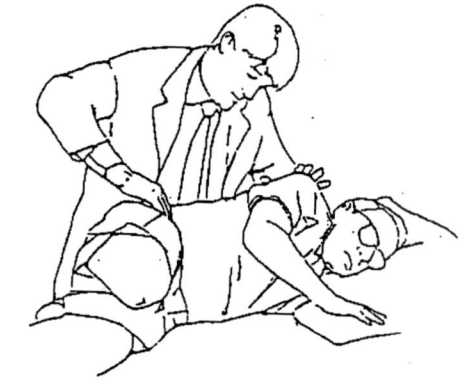

d. Command:
"Push your shoulder up and back and pull your pelvis up and forward." or "Twist into my hands"

Variation: If the therapist wants to promote stability through isometric contractions, the command: "Hold; don't let me move you" is employed while the therapist generates a force matching the patient's resistance.

Pattern: Anterior Trunk Rotation

a. Position:
Patient lies sidelying with hips and knees flexed to 90°, arms relaxed.

b. Manual contacts:
Distal hand - ischial tuberosity
Proximal hand - anterior aspect of the deltoid

c. Motion:
Trunk - anterior rotation
Shoulder girdle - anterior elevation
Pelvis - posterior depression

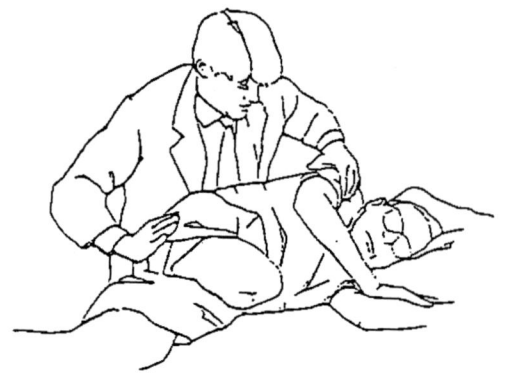

d. Command:
"Pull your shoulder up and forward and sit down and back." or
"Twist into my hands"

Variation: If the therapist desires to promote stability through isometric contractions, the command: "Hold; don't let me move you" is employed while the therapist generates a force matching the patient's resistance.

Traditional Lower Extremity Patterns

Pattern:
Flexion - Adduction - External Rotation (D1 fl)

a. Position:
   Patient lies supine.

b. Manual contacts:
   Distal hand - medial aspect of dorsum of foot
   Proximal hand - anterior/medial aspect of thigh proximal to patella

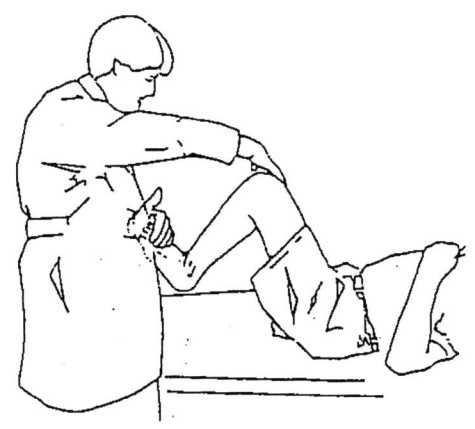

c. Motion:
   Hip: flex., add., ext. rot.
   Knee: flex.
   Ankle: dorsiflex., inver.

d. Command:
   "Pull your foot up and in."

Pattern:
Extension-Abduction-Internal Rotation (D1 ex)

a. Position:
   Patient lies supine.

b. Manual contacts:
   Distal hand - lateral aspect of plantar surface of foot.
   Proximal hand - posterior/lateral aspect of thigh to popliteal space.

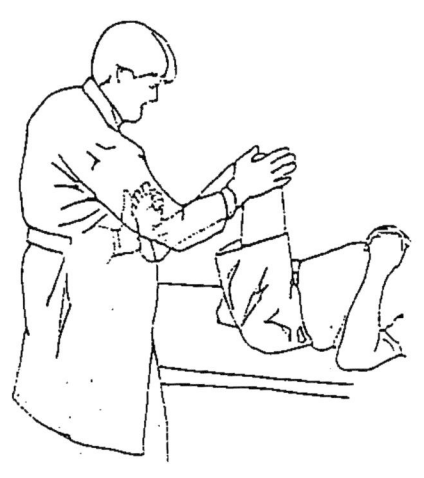

c. Motion:
   Hip: ext., abd., int. rot.
   Knee: ext.
   Ankle: plant. flex, ever.

d. Command:
   "Push your foot down and out."

Pattern:
Flexion-Abduction-Internal Rotation (D2 fl)

a. Position:
Patient lies supine.

b. Manual contacts:
Distal hand - lateral aspect of dorsum of foot.
Proximal hand - anterior/lateral aspect of thigh proximal to patella.

c. Motion:
Hip: flex., abd., int. rot.
Knee: flex.
Ankle: dorsiflex., ever.

d. Command:
"Pull your foot up and out."

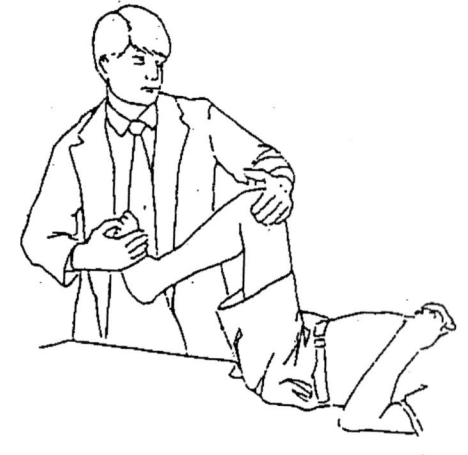

Pattern:
Extension-Adduction-External Rotation (D2 ex)

a. Position:
Patient lies supine.

b. Manual contacts:
Distal hand - medial aspect of plantar surface of foot.
Proximal hand - posterior/medial aspect of thigh proximal to popliteal space.

c. Motion:
Hip: ext., add., ext. rot.
Knee: ext.
Ankle: plantarflex., inver.

d. Command:
"Push your foot down and in."

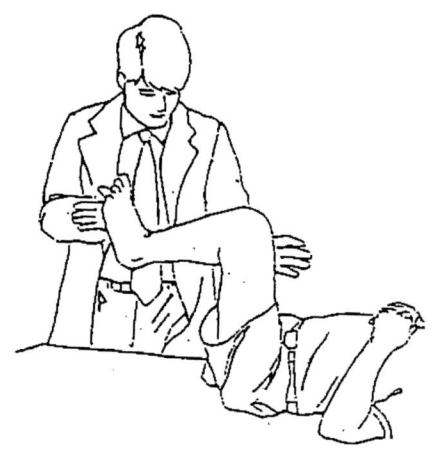

Lower Extremity Residual Limb Patterns

The following PNF extremity patterns are designed to be performed with amputees. Below-knee amputees require that the traditional manual contacts be moved proximally up the residual limb to accommodate the loss of the foot and ankle. If the length of the residual limb is too short, adopt the manual contacts used for above-knee amputees. Above-knee amputees require that both manual contacts be placed together, maintaining a lumbrical grip (MP flexion, and DIP, PIP extension). The rotational components at the hip may be more difficult to facilitate with the above-knee amputee because of the loss of leverage without a knee joint. Often, the femur will be too mobile within the soft tissue to promote significant rotation. If internal and external rotation are possible, consider this a bonus.

Pattern:
Flexion-Adduction-External Rotation (D1 fl)

a. Position:
Patient lies supine.

b. BKA manual contacts:
Distal hand - posterior/medial aspect of the distal residual limb.
Proximal hand - anterior/medial aspect of thigh proximal to patella.

AKA manual contacts:
Both hands - anterior/medial aspect of thigh proximal to the distal end.

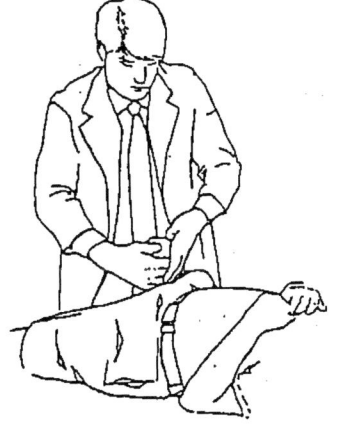

c. Motion:
Hip: flex., add., ext. rot.
Knee: flex.

d. Command:
"Pull your leg up and in."

Pattern:
Extension-Abduction-Internal Rotation (D1 ex)

a. Position:
Patient lies supine.

b. BKA manual contacts:
Distal hand - anterior/lateral aspect of the distal residual limb
Proximal hand - posterior/lateral aspect of thigh to popliteal space

AKA manual contacts:
Both hands - posterior/lateral aspect of thigh proximal to the distal end

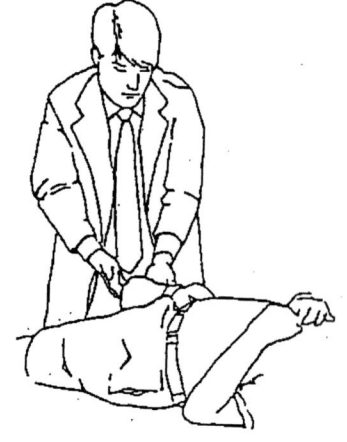

c. Motion:
Hip: ext., abd., int. rot.
Knee: ext.

d. Command:
"Push your leg down and out."

Pattern:
Flexion-Abduction-Internal Rotation (D2 fl)

a. Position:
Patient lies supine.

b. BKA manual contacts:
Distal hand - posterior/lateral aspect of the distal residual limb
Proximal hand - anterior/lateral aspect of thigh proximal to patella

AKA manual contacts:
Both hands - anterior/lateral aspect of thigh proximal to the distal end.

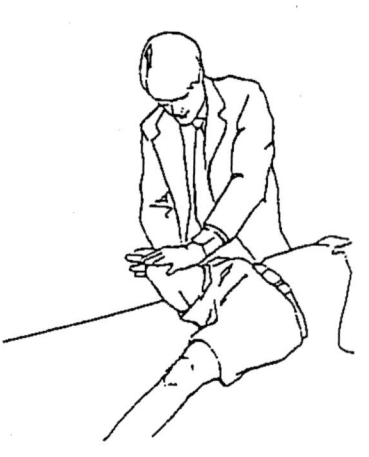

c. Motion:
Hip: flex., abd., int. rot.
Knee: flex.

d. Command:
"Pull your leg up and out."

Pattern:
Extension-Adduction-External Rotation (D2 ex)

a. Position:
   Patient lies supine.

b. BKA manual contacts:
   Distal hand - anterior/medial aspect of the distal residual limb.
   Proximal hand - posterior/medial aspect of thigh proximal to popliteal space.

   AKA manual contacts:
   Both hands - posterior/medial aspect of thigh proximal to the distal end.

c. Motion:
   Hip: ext., add., ext. rot.
   Knee: ext.

d. Command:
   "Push your leg down and in."

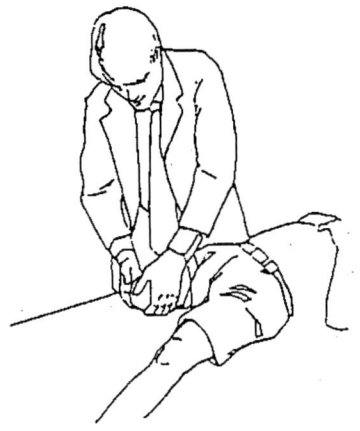

3. Isotonics [6, 9, 21, 24, 29]

Isotonic exercises require a dynamic contraction of the muscle which results in shortening or lengthening of the muscle as the joint moves throughout a predetermined range of motion.
The two types of contractions that result are:

1. <u>Concentric contraction</u> - Where the muscle shortens as it moves through the ROM. This is referred to as positive work, and permits acceleration of movement. A concentric contraction is typically employed when raising a weight or resistance.

2. <u>Eccentric contraction</u> - Where the muscle lengthens as it moves through the ROM. This is referred to as negative work, and permits deceleration of movement. An eccentric contraction is typically employed when lowering a weight or resistance.

A comparison of eccentric and concentric contractions demonstrates that a greater force is produced in an eccentric contraction. At comparable force levels, eccentric contractions require less motor unit activation as measured by EMG, and less cardiorespiratory response. However, muscle temperature, total heat production, cutaneous blood flow and muscle soreness are greater with eccentric contractions.

Advantages:
1. Optimally challenged with appropriate resistance, the muscle is given a higher intensity workout than provided with isometrics.
2. Both concentric and eccentric work are performed, creating the potential for greater strength gains than with isometric exercises.
3. Because movement about the joint is performed, ROM may be increased or at least maintained.
4. Many forms of isotonic exercise require joint stabilization and synergistic movements that promote muscular coordination.
5. As the ability to perform a greater number of repetitions and sets improves, so does muscular endurance.

Disadvantages:
1. Once weights and other equipment are introduced, the equipment cost and space requirements increase.
2. Often, supervision is required to ensure safety.
3. A higher risk of injury exists with weights and other equipment because of the potential for throwing the weights, dropping weights, and substitution of movement causing stress on related joints.
4. In order to move the baseline weight, a minimal strength level is required.
5. Often individuals must work at a sub-maximal intensity because of the inability of the resistance to accommodate to changes of muscle strength throughout the ROM.
6. Muscular soreness and fatigue are greater.
7. Greater irritation to degenerative and arthritic joints is possible.

Equipment
1. A large, firm, resting surface such as a floor or exercise mat. With some exercises, a chair may be appropriate.
2. Loose comfortable clothing, i.e. shorts and a T-shirt.
3. Towel roll of 5-7 inches in thickness and/or 2-4 pillows.
4. Cuff weights, rubber tubing, dumbbells or other weights.
5. Since the requirements for many of the individual exercises may vary, specific equipment needs for each exercise will be identified.

Suggested Techniques:[6,9,21,24,29]

When performing any isotonic exercise, whether the resistance is provided by gravity, manually, or with a weight, some form of cadence must be employed to derive maximum benefit from each repetition. The literature regarding isotonic exercise provides numerous protocols for strengthening, including various routines that vary in the prescribed cadence, as well as in the number of repetitions and sets to be performed.

Three of the most common methods of resistive isotonic strengthening have been repeatedly described in the literature: 1) Progressive Resisitive Exercise (PRE) Delorme method, Delorme (1951), 2) Oxford method, Zinovieff (1951) and 3) Daily Adjustable Progressive Resistive Exercise (DAPRE), Knight (1979). Each of the three programs work on a variation of the 10 repetition maximum principle, where 3-4 sets of 6-10 repetitions are performed with the resistance varying depending on the protocol and the individual's ability to lift a maximum weight for 6-10 repetitions. These time-tested methods have produced significant results in both healthy and debilitated individuals.

In an attempt to simplify what can be a very confusing issue, this text has elected to present a single protocol for isotonic strengthening. This is not to say that any one method is superior over another, but rather it is an attempt to reduce possible confusion for the reader. Therapists may elect to modify or alter the program presented to fit the individual needs of the amputee.

Eccentric contractions are stronger than concentric, and therefore, a heavier load or a longer duration of work is required to fatigue this type of contraction. Subsequently, the following cadence is offered as the standard for all the isotonic exercises described in this text. The concentric contraction should take 2 seconds to perform. At the peak of the movement, a 1 second pause should be taken to ensure control of the movement, followed by a 4 second eccentric contraction. The eccentric phase is twice as long as the concentric to promote fatigue of both types of contraction. If 8 to 12 repetitions are performed with each exercise, then the average number of repetitions will be 10. Therefore, if each repetition lasts for 7 seconds and an average of 10 repetitions are performed for a average total time of 70 seconds, then each exercise set will utilize the body's anaerobic energy system, which will assist in building muscle strength rather than muscular endurance.

The following program is presented as an active exercise program which is an excellent starting point for independent strengthening when progressing from isometrics exercises. After the amputee is able to perform 12 to 15 repetitions and has sufficiently mastered the active exercise program, resistive exercise should be introduced in order to further the strengthening process. The technique for the exercises remains the same, however, an appropriate succession of cuff weights, free weights, or incremented resistance of rubber tubing should be added to provide a progression to the resistive exercise program.

The exercises are described for the amputated limb, but it is recommended that the sound limb be included in all strengthening exercises to ensure maximum benefit, which will enhance performance of functional skills.

Precautions:
The two absolute indications for cessation of isotonics or resistive exercise are inflammation and pain. The signs and symptoms of inflammation include: swelling, heat, and redness around the joint. Exercise should be discontinued if pain, with or without movement, occurs either: 1) immediately during exercise as an acute pain, 2) lasts longer than 3 hours after exercise, or 3) 72 hours after exercise and does not present as delayed onset muscles soreness (DOMS).

Lower Extremity Strengthening
General Instructions:*

1. Strength training must be progressive. You should constantly attempt to increase the number of repetitions or the amount of resistance in every workout.

2. Perform 8-15 repetitions. Once 12-15 repetitions are performed correctly and safely, increase the weight by 5-10% (5lbs), or increase the resistance of the rubber tubing.

3. Each repetition consists of:
    2 second concentric contraction (raising phase)
    1 second pause at the peak of the movement
    4 second eccentric contraction (lowering phase)
    7 seconds for each repetition

4. Substitution or "jerky" movements should be avoided, as they are not conducive to progressive strength gains and may lead to possible injury.

5. All movements should be performed throughout the greatest available range of motion.

6. The order of exercise selection should progress from the largest and proceed down to the smallest muscle groups.

7. One set is usually all that is required for any one muscle group or exercise if 100% effort has been applied.

8. Each exercise session should never last more than one hour.

9. Strengthening should be performed every other day, or a minimum of three times per week.

10. An attempt to make the exercise program fun and interesting should be made avoiding a boring regimen that will soon be abandoned.

*Adapted from: Darden,E.: Strength training principles. Winter Park, FL, Anna Publishing, Inc. 1977.

Program example:
    10 repetitions
    x 7 seconds per repetition
    70 seconds
    x 15 exercises per session
    17 minutes 30 seconds
    2 minutes between each exercise
    45 minutes total exercise time

Precaution:
The non-exercised foot and leg, as well as the amputated leg, must be carefully observed and positioned so that no undue pressure is placed on any part of the limb causing friction that may result in a lesion. When using cuff weights or rubber tubing, extreme care must be taken not to cause abrasions to the skin while securing the resistive device to the limb or during exercise.

Warning: Any exercise activities not approved by appropriate medical personnel can have harmful results. Prior to starting any exercise program, have your doctor or therapist assess your medical and physical status. All exercise programs should be prescribed by a board-certified and registered professional. If, at any time, sudden pain or lasting discomfort should result, consult your doctor immediately.

1. Hip Flexion

   a. Lie on your back comfortably with both legs straight, both arms resting at your sides.

   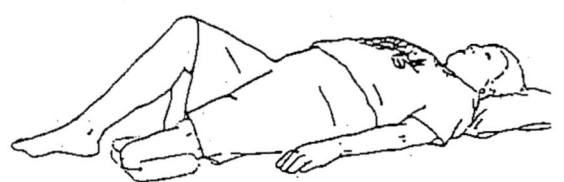

   Variation: A towel roll may be placed under the non-exercised knee to prevent low back strain.

   b. Raise your leg approximately 12 inches, for a count of _____ seconds.

   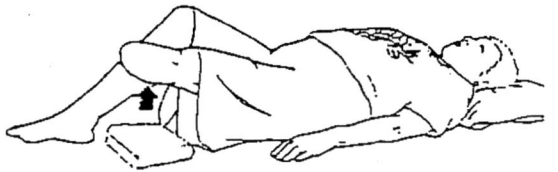

   c. Hold the raised position for a count of _____ second(s).

   d. Slowly lower your leg for a count of _____ seconds.

   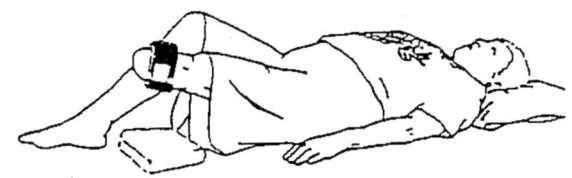

   e. Repeat for _____ repetitions, performing _____ sets.

   Primary muscles: abdominals, iliopsoas, and rectus femoris

2. Hip Abduction

   a. Lie on your side with both legs straight. One arm rests in front of you, the other arm under your head.

   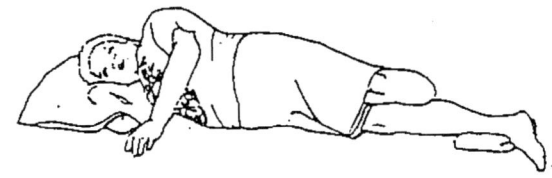

   Variation: When the residual limb is healing, place a pillow between your thighs. The sound limb knee may bend extending the leg behind you.

   b. Raise the upper leg approximately 12 inches, for a count of _____ seconds.

   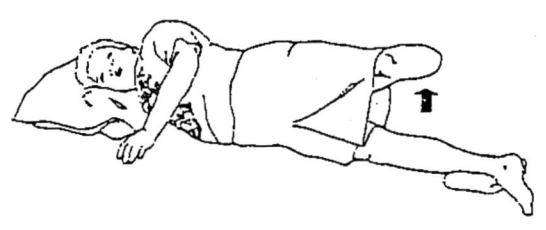

   c. Hold the raised position for a count of _____ second(s).

   d. Lower your leg for a count of _____ seconds.

   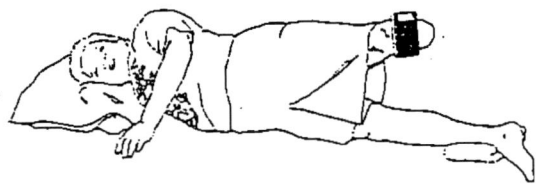

   e. Repeat for _____ repetitions, performing _____ sets.

   Primary muscles: gluteus medius, gluteus minimus, tensor fascia lata

3. Hip Adduction

   a. Lie on your side with the lower leg straight and the upper leg bent to 90 degrees at the hip and knee, resting on a pillow. The upper arm rests in front of you, the lower arm is tucked under your head.

   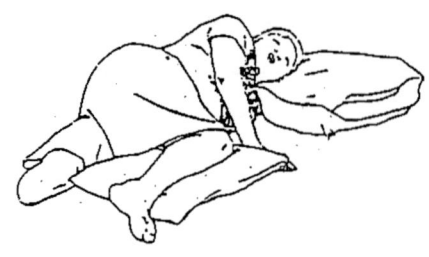

   b. Raise the lower leg approximately 6 inches, for a count of _____ seconds.

   c. Hold the raised position for a count of _____ second(s).

   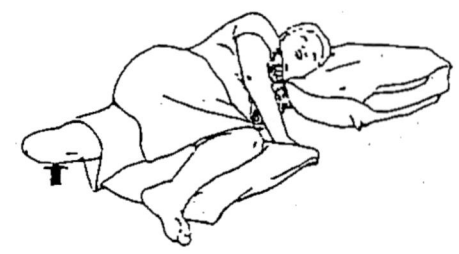

   d. Lower your leg for a count of _____ seconds.

   e. Repeat for _____ repetitions, performing _____ sets.

   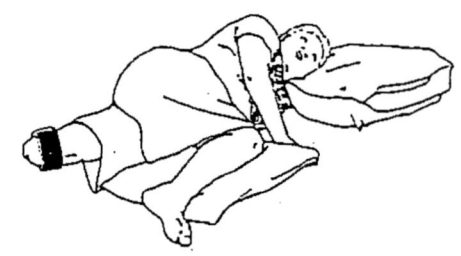

   Primary muscles: adductor magnus, adductor longus, adductor brevis and gracilis

4. Hip Extension

   a. Lie on your stomach with both legs straight. Both arms at your sides.

   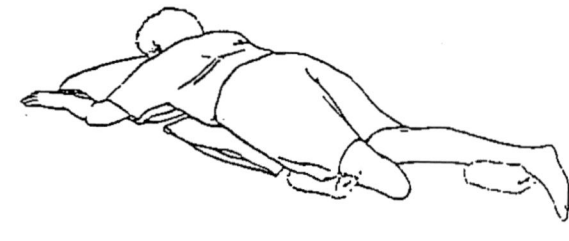

   Variation: A pillow may be placed under the hips to prevent low back strain. A towel pad may be placed under both thighs and the ankle to prevent excessive pressure.

   b. Raise your leg approximately 6 inches, for a count of _____ seconds.

   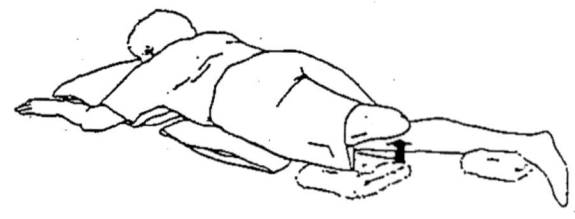

   c. Hold the raised position for a count of _____ second(s).

   d. Slowly lower your leg for a count of _____ seconds.

   e. Repeat for _____ repetitions, performing _____ sets.

   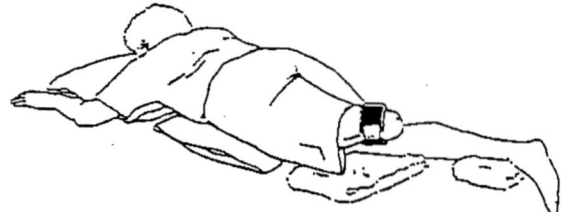

Primary muscles: gluteus maximus, hamstrings

5. Knee Flexion

   a. Lie on your stomach with both legs straight. Both arms rest at your sides

   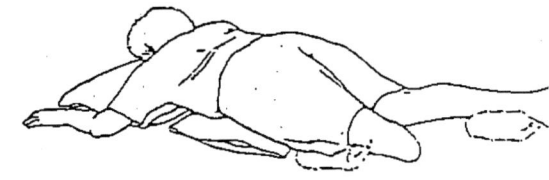

   Variation: A pillow may be placed under the hips to prevent low back strain. A towel pad may be place under both thighs and the ankle to prevent excessive pressure.

   b. Bend your knee for a count of _____ seconds, until your lower leg is perpendicular to the resting surface.

   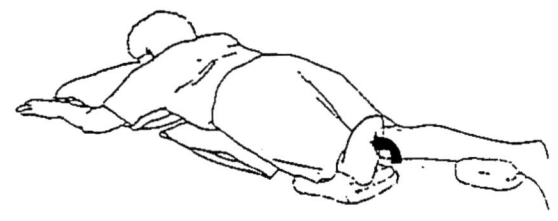

   c. Hold the raised position for a count of _____ second(s).

   d. Slowly lower your leg for a count of _____ seconds.

   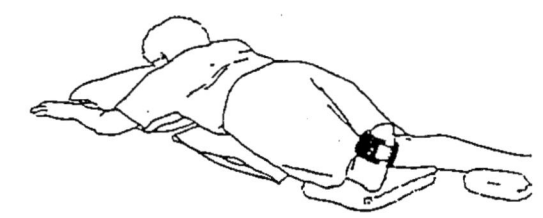

   e. Repeat for _____ repetitions, performing _____ sets.

   Primary muscles: hamstrings

6. Knee Extension

   a. Lie on your back with the sound limb straight, and a large towel roll under the knee of the residual limb.

   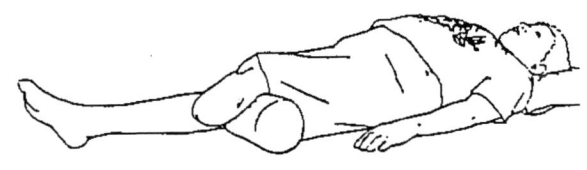

   Variation: Sitting upright on the edge of a chair, place a towel roll under your knee and permit your leg to hang freely toward the floor.

   b. Raise your leg, straightening the knee, for a count of _____ seconds.

   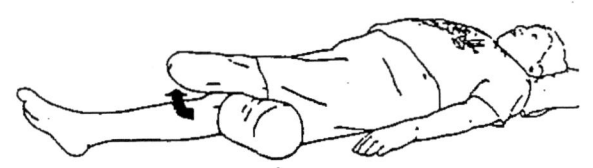

   c. Hold your leg in the raised position for a count of _____ second(s).

   d. Lower your leg for a count of _____ seconds.

   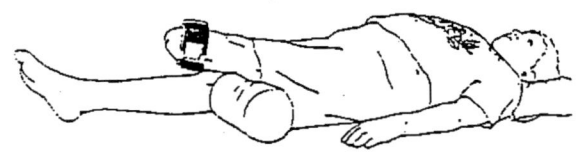

   e. Repeat for _____ repetitions, performing _____ sets.

   Primary muscles: quadriceps

7. Ankle Pumps

a. Lie on your back with both legs straight. Arms rest at your sides.

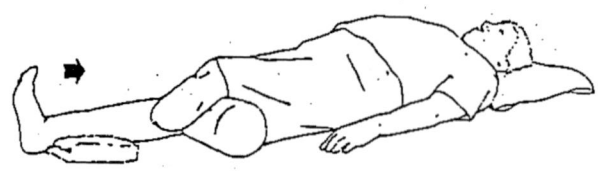

Variation: A towel roll may be placed under the non-exercised knee to prevent low back strain.

b. Pull your foot back as far as possible, and hold for a count of _____ seconds.

c. Next, point your foot down as far as possible, and hold for a count of _____ seconds.

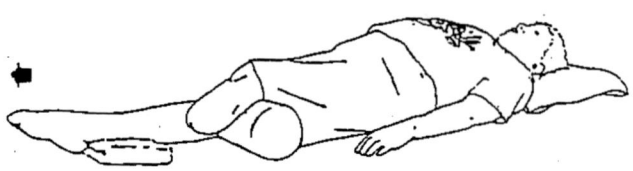

d. Alternate the upward/downward motions.

e. Repeat for _____ repetitions, performing _____ sets.

Primary muscles: ankle musculature

8. Half Sit-Ups

a. Lie on your back with pillows or a foam wedge under your shoulders. Cross your arms over your chest.

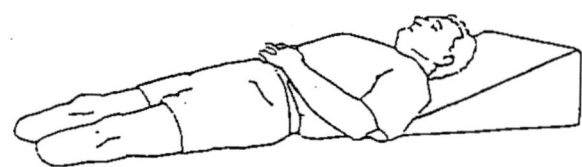

Variation: Your knee(s) may be slightly flexed, resting on a towel or bolster.

b. Gently tuck your chin toward your chest, continuing to raise your shoulders until your upper back is off the resting surface.

c. Hold the raised position for a count of _____ second(s).

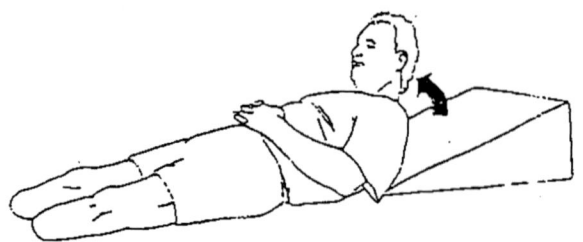

d. Lower your upper trunk and head down to the resting surface, for a count of _____ seconds.

e. Repeat for _____ repetitions, performing _____ sets.

page 46

Variation: Cross your arms behind your head for greater difficulty.

Primary muscles: upper abdominals

9. Abdominal Crunches

a. Lie on your back. Cross your arms over your chest.

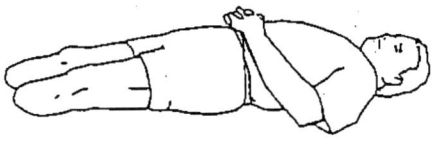

b. Simultaneously raise your head, shoulders, and legs until they are approximately 12 inches off the resting surface.

c. Hold the raised position for a count of _____ second(s).

d. Lower your upper trunk and legs down to the resting surface for a count of _____ seconds.

e. Repeat for _____ repetitions, performing _____ sets.

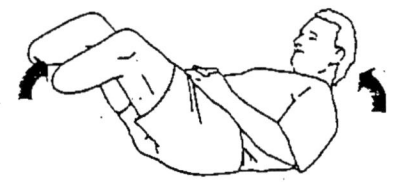

Variation: Cross your arms behind your head for greater difficulty.

Primary muscles: upper and lower abdominals, hip flexors

10. "The Walkermatic"

Equipment:
An adjustable Velcro strip is placed at the center of a walker frame with four pieces of surgical tubing tied at equal intervals attaching the Velcro strip to the walker. Surgical tubing may be added or subtracted to appropriately adjust the resistance.

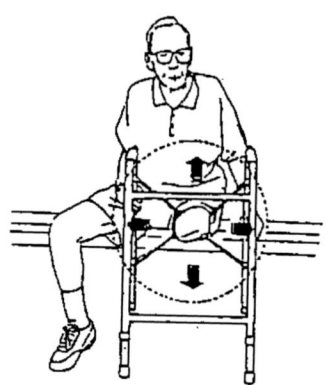

a. The patient sits on the edge of a mat, placing the walker in front of them. They may rest their hands on the walker for balance during the exercise.

b. The amputee performs one of the following: flexion, abduction, adduction, extension, for a count of _____ seconds.

c. Hold the position for a count of _____ second(s).

d. Return the residual limb to the center position for a count of _____ seconds.

e. Repeat for _____ repetitions, performing _____ sets.

Upper Extremity Strengthening

After amputation, the lower extremity amputee will initially require significant upper extremity strength in order to perform their activities of daily living (ADLs) from a wheelchair, or if appropriate, with the use of crutches or a walker. Sufficient upper extremity strength will allow the new amputee to be more independent during bathroom, tub, and bed transfers to the wheelchair, as well as during pre-prosthetic gait training.

Just as continued strengthening with weight machines or other forms of strength training are beneficial for the lower extremity, so are they equally beneficial for the upper extremity.

The principles outlined for isotonic exercises for lower extremities apply for upper extremity strengthening. Slow, deliberate movements throughout the available range of motion which avoid substitution, and allow for the weight to be controlled, are paramount to safely deriving the maximum benefit from each exercise.

The following exercises should be modified appropriately according to the amputee's medical condition, age, and initial strength assessment. All exercises should be performed on a firm resting surface, such as a mat table or the floor.

Equipment:
1. Dumbbells
2. Cuff weights
3. Surgical tubing
4. Soup cans in a pillow case

Warning: Any exercise activities not approved by appropriate medical personnel can have harmful results. Prior to starting any exercise program, have your doctor or therapist assess your medical and physical status. All exercise programs should be prescribed by a board-certified and registered professional. If, at any time, sudden pain or lasting discomfort should result, consult your doctor immediately.

Upper Extremity Strengthening
General Instructions:

1. Strength training must be progressive. You should constantly attempt to increase the number of repetitions or the amount of resistance in every workout.

2. Perform 8-15 repetitions. Once 12-15 repetitions are performed correctly and safely, increase the weight by 5-10% (5lbs), or increase the resistance of the rubber tubing.

3. Each repetition consists of:
    2 second concentric contraction (raising phase)
    1 second pause at the peak of the movement
    <u>4 second eccentric contraction (lowering phase)</u>
    7 seconds for each repetition

4. Substitution or "jerky" movements should be avoided, as they are not conducive to progressive strength gains and may lead to possible injury.

5. All movements should be performed throughout the greatest available range of motion.

6. The order of exercise selection should progress from the largest and proceed down to the smallest muscle groups.

7. One set is usually all that is required for any one muscle group or exercise if 100% effort has been applied.

8. Each exercise session should never last more than one hour.

9. Strengthening should be performed every other day, or a minimum of three times per week.

Program example:
    10 repetitions
    <u>x 7 seconds per repetition</u>
    70 seconds
    <u>x 15 exercises per session</u>
    17 minutes 30 seconds
    <u>2 minutes between each exercise</u>
    45 minutes total exercise time

1. Wheelchair Barbell Raise

   Equipment: The wheelchair barbell consists of two wheelchair wheels connected by a metal bar. The wheels should be fastened securely in place, and additional weights should be added as appropriate.

   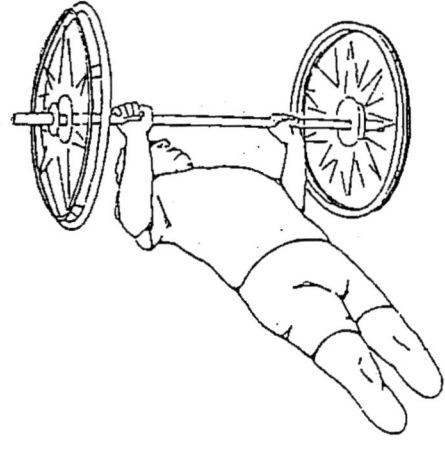

   a. Lie on your back with both legs straight. The "wheelchair barbell" is placed at chest level, hands placed shoulder width apart on the barbell, palms facing upward.

   b. Raise the barbell slowly for a count of _____ seconds, until the elbows are extended but not forcefully "locked out".

   c. Hold the extended position for a count of _____ second(s).

   d. Slowly lower the barbell for a count of _____ seconds.

   e. Repeat for _____ repetitions, performing _____ sets.

   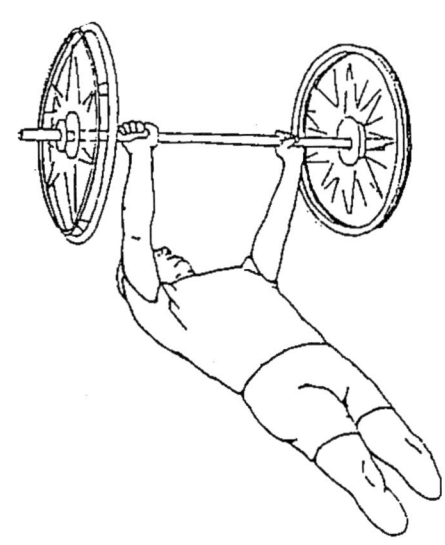

   Primary muscles: pectoralis major and minor, triceps

2. Shoulder Press

   a. Sitting upright on the edge of a mat or chair, gently grip the weights in each hand, with palms facing upward, elbows bent and hands at shoulder height.

   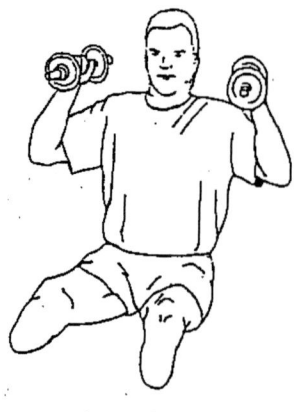

   b. Raise your arms, straightening (but not forcefully "locking out") your elbows over your head slowly, for a count of _____ seconds.

   c. Hold your arms in the raised position for a count of _____ second(s).

   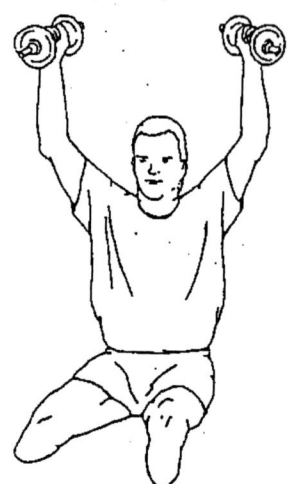

   d. Slowly lower the weights down to shoulder height for a count of _____ seconds.

   e. Repeat for _____ repetitions, performing _____ sets.

   Primary muscles: deltoids and triceps

3. Lateral Raises

   a. Sitting upright on the edge of a mat or chair, grip the weights in each hand, with palms facing inward, elbows bent at a 90 degree angle.

   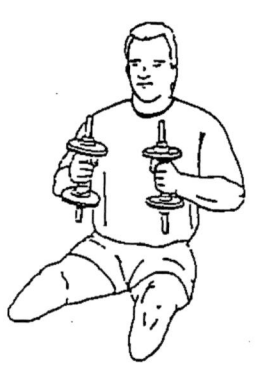

   b. Raise your arms slowly, for a count of _____ seconds, until your elbows and hands are equal height to your shoulders.

   c. Hold your arms in the raised position for a count of _____ second(s).

   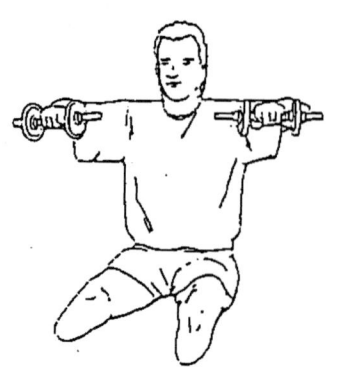

   d. Slowly lower the weights back down for a count of _____ seconds.

   e. Repeat for _____ repetitions, performing _____ sets.

Primary muscles: deltoids

4. Dips

Equipment: Blocks of various heights, small foot stools or a walker with shortened legs may be used. The greater the height of the block or stool, the more difficult the exercise. This exercise may also be performed in a wheelchair, using the armrests.

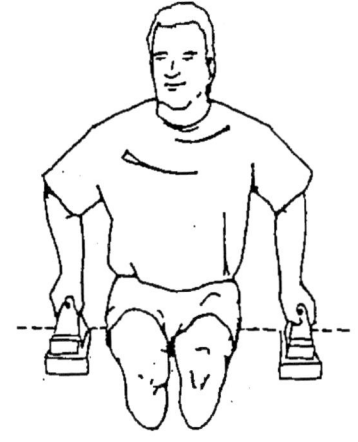

a. Sitting with both legs straight, place the dip blocks to either side of your hips while resting your hands comfortably on the top of the block surface.

b. Push downward into the block, straightening your elbows (but not forcefully "locking them out"), slowly raising your buttocks off the resting surface for a count of _____ seconds.

c. Hold the extended elbows position for _____ second(s).

d. Slowly lower yourself back to the resting surface for a count of _____ seconds.

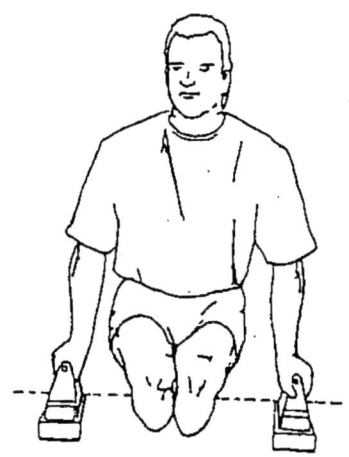

e. Repeat for _____ repetitions, performing _____ sets.

Variation: To increase the difficulty of the exercise, the lower extremities are raised off the mat simultaneously with the buttocks.

Primary muscles: triceps and deltoids

5. Elbow Flexion

a. Sitting upright on the edge of a mat or chair, grip the weights in each hand, with palms facing up, elbows straight.

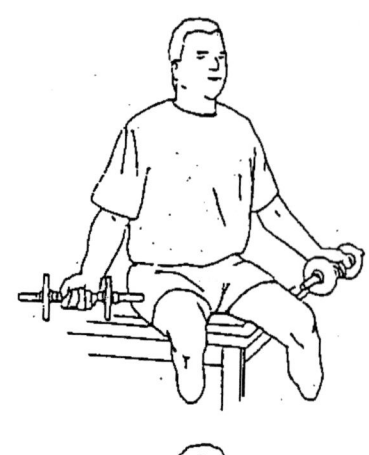

b. Bend your elbows, lifting the weights for a count of ____ seconds.

c. Hold the elbows in the bent position for a count of ____ second(s).

d. Slowly lower the weights back down for a count of ____ seconds.

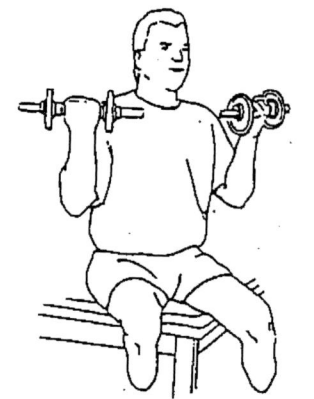

e. Repeat for ____ repetitions, performing ____ sets.

Primary muscles: biceps

6. Elbow Extension

a. Sitting upright on the edge of a mat or chair, gently grip the weights in both hands, bring both hands and the weight behind your head at shoulder level, elbows fully bent.

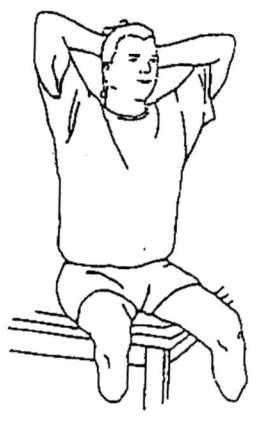

b. Raise the weights, straightening (but not forcefully "locking out") your elbows over your head, for a count of ____ seconds.

c. Hold your arms in the raised position for a count of ____ second(s).

d. Slowly lower the weights back down behind your head for a count of ____ seconds.

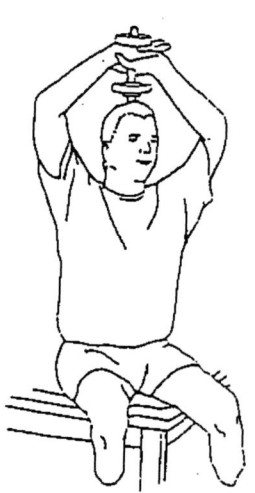

e. Repeat for ____ repetitions, performing ____ sets.

Primary muscles: triceps

7. Wrist Flexion

a. Sitting upright on the edge of a mat or chair, gently grip the weights in each hand, place your forearms on your thighs, palms upward, elbows bent at a 90 degree angle.

b. Raise the weights so that only your wrists bend, for a count of _____ seconds.

c. Hold your hands in the raised position for a count of _____ second(s).

d. Lower the weights down for a count of _____ seconds.

e. Repeat for _____ repetitions, performing _____ sets.

Primary muscles: wrist flexors

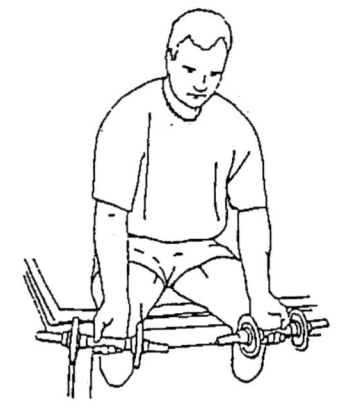

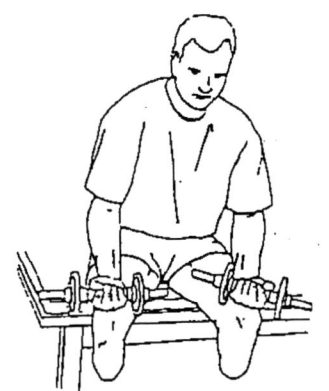

8. Wrist Extension

a. Sitting upright on the edge of a mat or chair, gently grip the weights in each hand, place your forearms on your thighs, palms downward, elbows bent at approximately a 90 degree angle.

b. Raise the weights so that only your wrists bend slowly, for a count of _____ seconds.

c. Hold your hands in the raised position for a count of _____ second(s).

d. Slowly lower the weights back down for a count of _____ seconds.

e. Repeat for _____ repetitions, performing _____ sets.

Primary muscles: wrist extensors

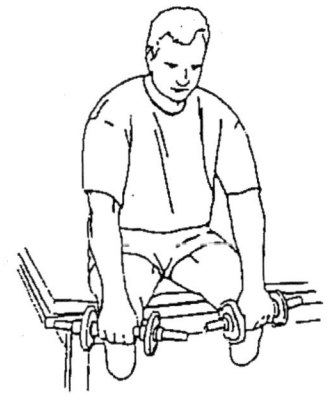

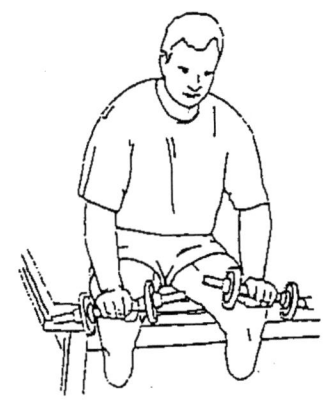

4. Isokinetics [7, 13, 17, 24]

Isokinetic exercise requires an isokinetic exercise device that presets the speed of movement performed by the muscle. The resistance applied to the muscle during either the concentric or eccentric contraction, is considered to be accomodating because it varies, and is dependent upon the force generated by the muscle as the limb moves through the range of motion.

It is important to keep in mind that both below- and above-knee amputees may benefit from isokinetic strengthening if a few modifications are made from the set-up traditionally used for non-amputee patients. Remember, there is no age limitation placed upon isokinetic exercise. If an amputee is an appropriate candidate, isokinetics should be considered.

Advantages:
1. Multiple types of muscular contractions may be performed depending on the capabilities of the isokinetic device. (concentric, eccentric or isometric)
2. Safety- the resistance applied is dependent upon the effort put forth by the patient. There are no pre-determined weights to overcome or drop.
3. The accomodating resistance permits the muscle to work at an optimal level throughout the entire range of motion.
4. The speed control allows the muscle to perform at a variety of velocities.
5. When exercising at the higher speeds, there is a decrease in the joint compressive forces. This is a significant advantage for patients with articular cartilage pathology.

Disadvantages:
1. Isokinetic devices are expensive.
2. The availability of the isokinetic devices is limited in the clinical setting, and trained supervision is required.
3. Generally, only one patient and one joint can utilize the equipment at a time.
4. The strength reports generated from each different brand of isokinetic device vary. Therefore, there is no universal consistency in the strength values reported between the various brands of isokinetic devices.

Equipment:

Because each isokinetic device provides different options, in terms or speed of motion, types of exercises, patient set-up and information provided to the operator, the specifics of equipment cannot be discussed in this text. The principles and exercise protocols for isokinetic strengthening have been well outlined in the literature.

General Instructions:

Gould and Davies (1985), suggest a progression of strengthening exercises for isokinetic strengthening that includes sub-maximal and maximal; multiple-angle isometric, short-arc and full ROM exercises. Each type of strengthening program selected is dependent upon the patient's level of rehabilitation. For example, the patient would begin with sub-maximal multiple-angle isometrics (isometrics performed at a series of different angles, 20° apart) and progress to maximal isometrics. The progression would continue onto submaximal short arc (partial ROM) exercise to maximal short-arc to submaximal and finally maximal full ROM resistive exercise.

The purpose of limiting ROM is to prevent further injury to an injured joint or to a post-surgical limb. If the amputee has full ROM and the joint is not compromised, strengthening should be done throughout the complete range.

The following figures illustrate two methods of strength training with isokinetic devices. Figure 1. is a representation of multiple-angle isometrics performed at 20° apart for both the knee and hip flexion, and extension. The speed of the isokinetic device is set to zero and the resistance arm is set for the appropriate joint angle. The Rule of Ten is applied. [25]

Figure 1. Knee and hip flexion/extension multiple-angle isometric positions.

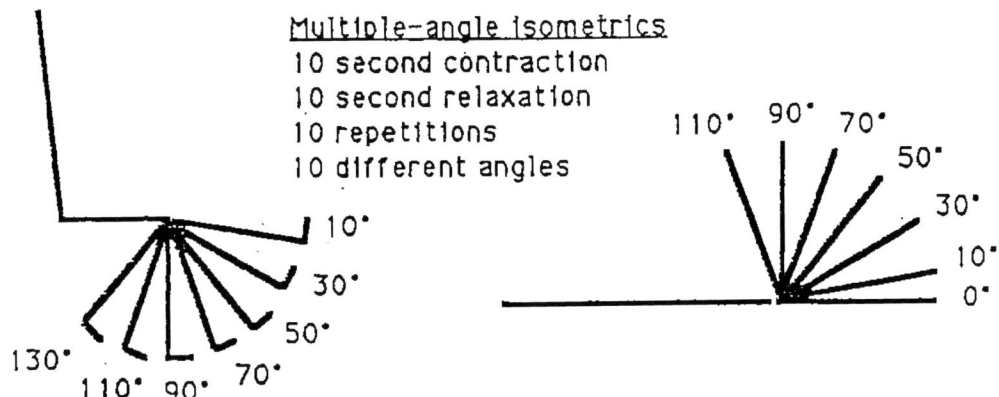

One strengthening program that requires concentric contractions throughout the available ROM is the Velocity Spectrum Rehabilitation Protocol (VSRP). This program identifies pre-selected repetitions over a series of speeds. The examples in figure 2. illustrate a slow speed and high speed VSRP model. The numerals represent speed in degrees per second. If 10 repetitions are performed at each speed, then given the 10 sets, a total of 100 repetitions would be performed for each VSRP. [7]

Figure 2. VSRP training program for slow and fast speeds.

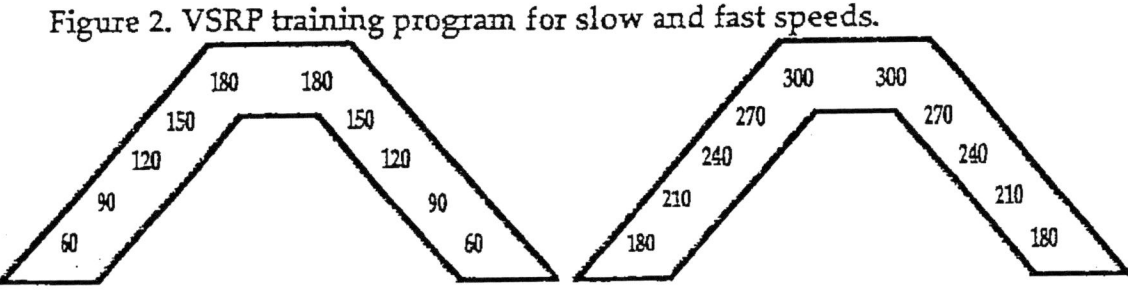

Slow Speed VSRP   High Speed VSRP

Adapted from: Davies GJ, "Compendium of isokinetics in clinical usage" S&S Publishers, Onalska, WI, 1992

1. Hip Abduction/Adduction

   a. The patient lies in sidelying on a plinth or bench with the amputated side uppermost; the dynamometer aligned to the hip joint. The residual limb is attached appropriately to the resistance arm.

   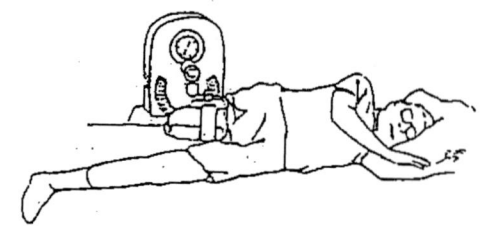

   b. Abduct and adduct the hip at the appropriate speed and for the number of repetitions for the selected strength training protocol.

   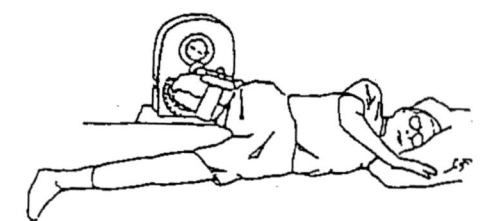

   c. Rest the limb for _____ seconds between the exercise sets.

   d. Perform _____ sets.

2. Hip Flexion/Extension

   a. The patient lies supine on a plinth or bench; the dynamometer is aligned to the hip joint. The residual limb is attached appropriately to the resistance arm.

   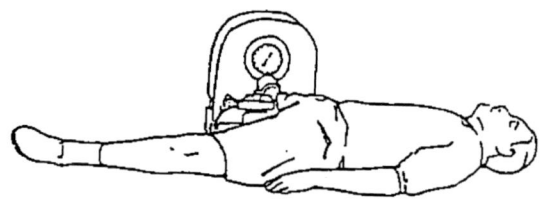

   b. Flex and extend the hip at the appropriate speed and for the number of repetitions for the selected strength training protocol.

   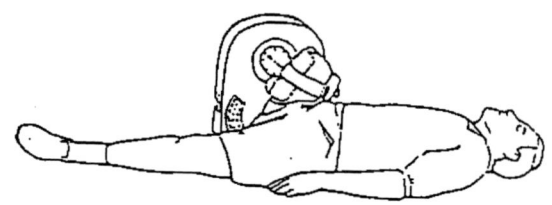

   c. Rest the limb for _____ seconds between the exercise sets.

   d. Perform _____ sets.

3. Knee Flexion/Extension

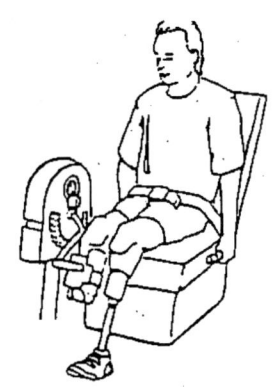

a. The patient sits on the seat of the isokinetic device. The residual limb is attached to the arm, with padding or other modifications as needed for comfort and appropriate support.

b. Flex and extend the knee at the appropriate speed and for the number of repetitions for the selected strength training protocol.

c. Rest the limb for _____ seconds between the exercise sets.

d. Perform _____ sets.

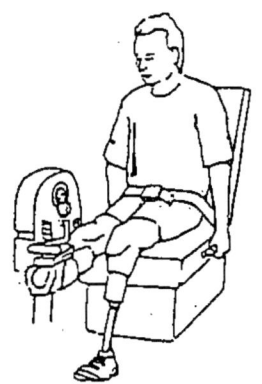

References

1. Anderson, JE: Grant's Atlas of Anatomy. 8th ed, William and Wilkins Baltimore; 1983.

2. Anderson MH, Bechtol CO, Sollars RE: Clinical Prosthetics for Physicians and Therapists. Springfield, Illinois: Charles C. Thomas Publisher; 1959.

3. Banerjee SN, (ed.) Rehabilitation Management of Amputees. Baltimore, MD, Williams and Wilkins; 1982.

4. Basmajian JV, Muscles Alive: Their Function Revealed by Electromyography. Baltimore, MD, Williams and Wilkins Co; 1978.

5. Bowker, JH, Michaels, JW, (ed) AAOS Atlas of Limb Prosthetics: Surgical, Prosthetic, and Rehabilitation Principles. St. Louis, MO, Mosby Year Book; 1992.

6. Darden, E: Strength Training Principles. Winter Park, FL Anna Publishing, Inc; 1977.

7. Davies, GJ: A Compendium of Isokinetics in Clinical Usage and Rehabilitation Techniques. 2nd ed. La Crosse, WI, S&S Publishing; 1985.

8. Davies GJ, Ellenbecker TS, Eccentric Isokinetics. Orthop Phys Ther Clin of N Amer. 1992; 1:297

9. DeLorme, TL, Watkins, AL: Progressive Resistive Exercise: Technic and Medical Application. New York, NY, Appleton-Century-Crofts, Inc; 1951.

10. Eisert O, Tester O W: Dynamic exercises of lower extremity amputees. Arch Phys Med Rehabil. 1954; 35:695

11. Engstrom B, Van de Van C: Physiotherapy For Amputees The Roehampton Approach. New York, NY, Churchill Livingston; 1985.

12. Gailey RS, Gailey AM: Prosthetic Gait Training Program for Lower Extremity Amputees. Miami, FL, Advanced Rehabilitation Therapy, Inc; 1992.

13. Gould, JA, Davies GJ: Orthopaedic and Sports Physical Therapy. St. Louis, MO, CV Mosby Co; 1985.

14. Gossman M, Sahrmann S, Rose S, Review of length-associated changes in muscle. Phys Ther 1982; 62:1799

15. Gross M: Intra-machine and inter-machine reliability of the Biodex and Cybex II for knee flexion and extension peak torque and angular work, J Orthop Sport Phys Ther. 1991; 13:329

16. Hallum, A and Medeiros, JM: Effect of duration of passive stretch on hip abduction range of motion. J Orthop Sports Phys Ther. 1987; 8:409

17. Hislop HJ, Perrine JJ: The isokinetic conept of exercise. Phys Ther. 1967; 47:114

18. Karacoloff L A: Lower Extremity Amputation A Guide to Functional Outcomes in Physical Therapy Management. Rockville, MD, Aspen Publication; 1986.

19. Kegel B, Burgess E M, Starr T W, Daly W K: Effects of isometric muscle training on residual limb volume, strength, and gait of below-knee amputees. Phy Ther. 1981; 61: 1419

20. Kendall, HD. Kendall, F.P. and Wadsworth, GE: Muscle Testing and Function, Baltimore, MD, William and Wilkins; 1983.

21. Kerr D, Brunnstrom S: Training of the Lower Extremity Amputee. Springfield, IL: Charles C. Thomas; 1956.

22. Kerstein M D, Zimmer H, Dugdale F E, Lerner E: Rehabilitation after bilateral lower extremity amputation. Arch Phys Med Rehabil. 1975; 56: 309

23. Kessler R, Hertling d., Management of Common Musculoskeletal Disorders. Philadelphia, PA, Harper Row; 1983.

24. Kisner, C, Colby, LA, Therapeutic exercise: foundations and techniques 2nd ed, Philadelphia,, PA, FA Davis; 1990.

25. Knapik, JJ, Mawadsley, RH, Ramos, MU: Angula. Specificity and test-mode specificity of isometric and isokinetic strength training. J Orthop Sports Phys Ther. 1983; 5:58

26. Knight KL: Knee rehabilitation by the daily adjustable progressive resistance exercise technique. Am J Sports Med. 1979; 7:336

27. Malone JM, Moore W, Leal JM, Childers S J: Rehabilitation for lower extremity amputation. Arch Surg. 1981; 116: 93

28. Medeiros J, Smidt G, Burmeister L et al, The influence of isometric exercise and passive stretch on hip joint motion. Phys Ther. 1977; 57:518

29. Mensch G, Ellis P: Physical Therapy Management of Lower Extremity Amputations. Rockville, MD: Aspen Publishing; 1986.

30. O'Sullivan SB, Cullen KE, Schmitz TJ: Physical Rehabilitation: Evaluation and Treatment Procedures. Philadelphia, PA, F.A. Davis Co; 1981.

31. Sanders GT: Lower Limb Amputations: A Guide to Rehabilitation. Philidelphia, PA, F.A. Davis Co; 1986.

32. Sullivan, PE, Markos, PD, Minor, MAD: An Intergrated Approach to Therapeutic Exercise: Therory and Clinical Application. Reston, VA, Reston Publishing Co; 1982.

33. Voss, DE, Ionta, MK, Beverly, MJ: Proprioceptive Neuromuscular Facilitation: Patterns and Techniques. 3rd ed., Philadelphia, PA, Harper & Row Publishers, Inc; 1985.

34. Zinovieff, AN: Heavy resistance exercise, the Oxford technique. Br J Phys Med. 1951; 14:129

ADVANCED REHABILITATION THERAPY, INC.

The *Functional Training Series* set of DVDs is designed to offer the most comprehensive strategies in amputee rehabilitation for physical therapists, prosthetists, and clients. The emphasis is on the ability to move quickly and smoothly while developing balance and stability. The biomechanics and training principles of basic running for amputees are also featured.

Functional Training Series titles available:

V-1	Functional Prosthetic Training Transtibial	$34.95 each
V-2	Functional Prosthetic Training Transfemoral	$34.95 each
V-3	Essentials of Amputee Running	$34.95 each
V-4	Biomechanics of Amputee Running	$34.95 each
V-5	Functional Training Series-4 DVD set	$125.00 set

The *Rehabilitation Series* set of DVDs and manuals are designed as instructional tools for rehabilitation professionals. The DVDs provide a detailed visual presentation of material covered in the manuals.

Rehabilitation Series titles available:

Prosthetic Gait Training	A105 DVD $24.95 each	A108	Manual $10.50 each
Stretching & Strengthening	A106 DVD $24.95 each	A109	Manual $10.50 each
Balance, Agility, Coordination	A107 DVD $24.95 each	A110	Manual $10.50 each
A112 Rehab Series-3 DVD set	$60.00		
A118 Rehab Series-3 Manual Set	$30.00		

Shipping: $7.75 first item and $2.50 each additional item. One set=one item. Outside the USA, please call or email for shipping cost. Purchase orders must be emailed, faxed, or mailed. Thank you.

Name_____ E-mail_____
Address_____ Ste/Apt_____
City_____ State_____ Zip Code_____ Phone_____
Visa/MC#_____ Exp Date_____ Check/PO#_____

Quantity   Item   Unit Price   Total Cost

_____
_____

Send order to: Order Total_____
Advanced Rehab Therapy, Inc   FL Residents add 7% tax_____
7641 SW 126 St   Shipping_____
Miami, FL 33156   Amount enclosed_____
Phone: 305.378.0855 Email: gaileyann@gmail.com
www.advancedrehabtherapy.com   Prices effective 7/1/2013